D1000440

Springer Series on MEDICAL EDUCATION

Series Editor: Steven Jonas, M.D.
Series Advisers: Howard S. Barrows, M.D. • John Gordon Freymann, M.D. •
David Rabin, M.D., M.P.H.

Arthur Kaufman, M.D., is Professor of Family, Community, and Emergency Medicine; Director of Family Medicine; and a Director of the Primary Care Curriculum at the University of New Mexico School of Medicine. He has pioneered the development of health services for needy groups including sex assault victims, prison inmates, and the homeless, and has published extensively in these areas. He is the recipient of local and national awards for his teaching and his innovative work in medical education.

Implementing Problem-Based Medical Education

Lessons from Successful Innovations

Arthur Kaufman, M.D.

Editor

Foreword by Hilliard Jason, M.D. Ed.D.

Springer Publishing Company
New York

Copyright © 1985 by Springer Publishing Company, Inc.

All rights reserved

No part of this publication may be reproduced, stored in a retrieval system, or transmitted in any form or by any means, electronic, mechanical, photocopying, recording, or otherwise, without the prior permission of Springer Publishing Company, Inc.

Springer Publishing Company, Inc.
536 Broadway
New York, New York 10012

85 86 87 88 89 / 5 4 3 2 1

Library of Congress Cataloging-in-Publication Data

Main entry under title:
Implementing problem-based medical education.
  (Springer series on medical education; v. 9)
  Includes bibliographies and index.
  1. Medicine Clinical—Study and teaching.   2. Medical sciences—Study and teaching.
3. Medical logic—Study and teaching.   4. Educational innovations.   5. University of New Mexico. School of Medicine. Primary Care Curriculum.   I. Kaufman, Arthur.   II. University of New Mexico. School of Medicine. Primary Care Curriculum.   III. Series: Springer series on medical education; 9. [DNLM: 1. Curriculum.   2. Education, Medical—New Mexico.   3. Learning.   4. Problem Solving.   5. Teaching—methods. W1 SP685SE v.9 / W 18 I34]
R834.I46 1986   610'.7'11   85-12707
ISBN 0-8261-4660-0

Printed in the United States of America

Contents

Contributors

Max D. Bennett, Ph.D., is Associate Professor of Family, Community and Emergency Medicine, the Planning Officer at the University of New Mexico Medical Center, and Director of Phase IB of the Primary Care Curriculum at the University of New Mexico School of Medicine.

Samuel W. Bloom, Ph.D., is Professor of Sociology and Community Medicine at the Mount Sinai School of Medicine and the Graduate School of the City University of New York. At Mount Sinai, he is Director, Division of Behavioral Sciences of the Department of Community Medicine.

Cooley Butler, M.D., is Associate Professor of Pathology and responsible for the Primary Care Curriculum Pathology program at the University of New Mexico School of Medicine.

Joan E. Christy, M.S., was educational coordinator of the Primary Care Curriculum program during its first five years of development and implementation. She now coordinates clinical problem-oriented learning and faculty development activities at the Texas College of Osteopathic Medicine.

Aleksandra Counsellor, M.S., is the Program Specialist for the Preceptorship Program, Department of Family, Community and Emergency Medicine, University of New Mexico School of Medicine.

Stewart Duban, M.D., is Associate Professor of Pediatrics, Head of its Child Development Section, and Director of Clinical Skills in the Primary Care Curriculum at the University of New Mexico School of Medicine.

William R. Galey, Ph.D., is Professor, Department of Physiology and chairman of the Tutorial and Curriculum Committee of the Primary Care Curriculum at the University of New Mexico School of Medicine.

Rebecca Jackson, M.D., is Assistant Professor of the Department of Family, Community and Emergency Medicine and has been involved with tutoring and tutor training in the Primary Care Curriculum since its inception.

Martin P. Kantrowitz, M.D., is Associate Professor of the Department of Family, Community and Emergency Medicine at the University of New Mexico School of Medicine, where he is also Assistant Dean of Community Professional Education. Prior to his current appointment, he served as the Chief Medical Officer of the National Health Service Corps in Washington, D.C.

Diane J. Klepper, M.D., is Associate Professor, Department of Medicine, Assistant Dean for Admissions and Student Affairs and Phase III Director of the Primary Care Curriculum at the University of New Mexico School of Medicine.

Susan M. Lucero is a Program Specialist III with the Primary Care Curriculum at the University of New Mexico School of Medicine. Ms. Lucero coordinates many aspects of the program's tutorial and curricular development.

Nancy Martinez-Burrola is a Program Specialist III in the Primary Care Curriculum, University of New Mexico School of Medicine. Ms. Martinez-Burrola coordinates many aspects of PCC's research, student evaluation, and international programs.

Stewart P. Mennin, Ph.D., is Associate Professor of Anatomy and Associate Director of the Primary Care Curriculum at the University of New Mexico School of Medicine.

Maggi Moore-West, Ph.D., is Assistant Professor of Family, Community and Emergency Medicine and Psychiatry and Coordinator of the Longitudinal Project in Medical Education at the University of New Mexico School of Medicine.

Diana E. Northup, M.S.L.S., is the Coordinator of the Simulated Patient Program for the Primary Care Curriculum and co-author of the *Information Searching Guides*. Formerly she was Chief of Education and Instruction Programs at the Medical Center Library, University of New Mexico.

S. Scott Obenshain, M.D., is Professor of Pediatrics, Assistant Dean of Undergraduate Medical Education and a Director of the Primary Care Curriculum at the University of New Mexico, School of Medicine.

Michael J. O'Donnell, Ph.D., is Assistant to the Dean of Education, Head Administrator of Biomedical Communications and a Clinical Psychologist at the University of New Mexico School of Medicine. He serves as an evaluation and educational consultant to the Primary Care Curriculum.

Kathleen Saunders, M.S., M.L.S., is Assistant Director, Educational Services at the University of New Mexico Medical Center Library. She was formerly a resource librarian for the Department of Family and Community Medicine, University of Massachusetts Medical School.

Berthold E. Umland, M.D., is Associate Professor of Family, Community and Emergency Medicine and the Director of the Family Practice Residency at the University of New Mexico. He is Chairman of the Steering II Committee, the overseeing body for all students in their clinical years.

J. Dayton Voorhees, M.D., is in the practice of Family Medicine in Corrales, New Mexico, and is Adjunct Assistant Professor of Family, Community and Emergency Medicine at the University of New Mexico School of Medicine. Formerly, he was coordinator of Phase IB of the Primary Care Curriculum at the University of New Mexico School of Medicine.

Robert E. Waterman, Ph.D., is Professor of Anatomy and Biology and Chairman of the Primary Care Curriculum Educational Policy Committee at the University of New Mexico School of Medicine.

Donald A. West, M.D., is Associate Professor and Director of Medical Student Education in Psychiatry and Chairperson of the Evaluation Committee, Primary Care Curriculum, University of New Mexico School of Medicine. He is Chairman of the Steering I Committee, the overseeing body for all students in their preclinical years.

Foreword

Following the Flexner-induced "shake-out" of the proprietary and marginal medical schools in this country, the process of medical education remained strikingly homogeneous for more than half a century. Until the 1960s, it was reasonable to imagine a medical student moving between almost any two schools in this country, while hardly skipping a beat.

Although shifts in fashion and funding patterns brought alterations in some organizational and scheduling features, these changes tended to move in waves, spreading among most medical schools of the country like an infection. Despite the complexity, importance, and cost of medical education, the process of educational design remained a learn-as-you-go enterprise, involving more tinkering than substance. Almost no funds or efforts were expended on systematic research and development on the process of medical education. Decision making was almost always a matter of those with the most local political influence exercising their best judgments, or, to be more precise, if less charitable, asserting their intuitive guesses and personal opinions.

In the 1960s, the U.S. Congress adopted the view that this country faced a serious shortage of physicians. Thus began an unprecedented—and probably never to be repeated—major infusion of government funding for the substantial expansion of existing medical schools and for the addition of more than 30 new medical schools. In less than two decades, this country's annual number of medical graduates increased by more than 75 percent. This quantitative explosion brought with it many efforts to effect qualitative changes in conventional medical education. One of the late entrants in that era's spirit of change was the so-called Primary Care Curriculum (PCC) at the University of New Mexico School of Medicine, the program that is the subject of this book.

Now that special funding support for educational expansion has disappeared, many of the accompanying educational explorations of the 1960s and 1970s are vanishing. Much of the sameness of the prior era is returning to the medical education landscape. Happily for those of us who worry about the long-term risks associated with institutional conformity and stagnation, not to mention those of us who are bothered by the drabness of conventional medical education, a few shining lights remain.

The process whereby most medical education evolves is less than intellectually satisfying. It lacks a systematic rationale and does not reflect careful planning. This book is a window on one of the few genuine beacons currently available in medical education. It provides a major step toward an intellectually rigorous conceptualization of the process and procedures of an appealing and effective alternative approach to designing and offering medical education.

This is a book about the origins, design, implementation, and effects of the PCC. It is also much more. It is a first-person account of a moving human experience, in which some deeply caring people search for ways to provide a humane, effective learning experience for students who are seen as preparing to be practitioners of a humane, changing profession.

Among many others things, the authors provide a splendid illustration of a fundamental principle of human growth: people are shaped at least as much by how they are treated as by what they are told. In conventional medical education, much of what we do produces unintended consequences, "side-effects." We do not set out intentionally to cause students to dislike the basic sciences or to have difficulty taking initiative in their own learning or to be deceptive about their own limitations. Yet for many students in many medical schools, these are among the side-effects of the ways they are treated. Unfortunately, many medical schools are not exempt from Marshall McLuhan's discomforting but insightful observation, "most institutions end up preventing the purposes for which they were created."

Part of the problem in learning medicine in conventional settings is nicely summarized in David Rogers' graphic image: adapting to conventional instruction is "like trying to drink water from a fire hose." This vivid characterization of the information overload to which medical students are typically subjected suggests part of the solution that is needed.

We need to give students more control of the pace at which they receive information. But even if our schools became places that could be depicted as offering an array of gentle, individually controlled water fountains, we must still deal with the next step: What happens after the information enters the system? Healthy bodies are well equipped to metabolize water, automatically extracting what is needed and discarding the rest. Unfortunately, we are not similarly endowed with inherent physiologic mechanisms for digesting information and experiences.

The capacity to learn effectively must be learned. The designers of the PCC have sought to have a positive impact on the continuing evolution of their students' skills as learners. They set out to explore the possibility that much could be gained by treating students differently from the ways in which students are treated in conventional settings. They sought, among other goals, to help medical students become eager, competent learners, who are open about their learning needs and skilled at pursuing them. They approached these goals, in part, through structural changes in the educational arrangements of the first two years of medical school (by using, for example, small tutorial groups and an extended community-based preceptorship) and partly through procedural changes (by using, for example, clinical problems as springboards to basic science learning and by creating an atmosphere that was maximally free of harsh feedback). An intriguing situation evolved. Most of the existing, rather conventional medical school was left largely untouched. A separate track was created for nearly one-third of the students, who participate in the PCC during their first two years.

Some striking contrasts have emerged, perhaps none more poignant than the observation that some of the conventional-track students have come to see the PCC students as "brown-nosers," as "too eager to please." This is a sad but vivid reminder of a worrisome problem in medical education. In conventional settings, many students are prone to seeing learning as something that is done to impress others. Many of the PCC students achieve the desirable, contrasting perspective of seeing their learning of medicine as a deeply personal goal. The evidence presented here of an approach to instruction that helps medical students feel a genuine sense of "ownership" of their own learning is one of this book's powerful messages.

One might imagine that having two contrasting educational postures within the same school would present the makings for a classic "shoot-out." This arrangement brings into sharp focus the differences between those who cling to the approaches that have come to be regarded as "conventional" and those who are urging the need for reform. This seems like a setup for oversimplified dichotomies and for battle lines to be drawn: Authoritarian vs. Collaborative; Controlling vs. Permissive; Harsh vs. Benevolent; Hard vs. Soft; Strong vs. Weak; Old vs. New. Yet, perhaps paradoxically, one of the important messages from the story told and the findings presented in this book may be that the demarcations are not that clear-cut. With time and careful effort, the shared wish for excellence at this school seems to be emerging as stronger than the rivalry over which approach to that goal is best.

The authors have managed to strike a nice balance between enthusiasm for their own creation and an openness to constructive self-

Acknowledgments

This book describes a collaborative effort by the students, staff, and faculty at the University of New Mexico School of Medicine who worked diligently over the past seven years to create a different approach to medical education—the Primary Care Curriculum (PCC).

Perhaps the major credit for this work rests with the vision and faith shown in the University of New Mexico School of Medicine by the Kellogg Foundation that gave so generously to PCC's development. Andrew Patullo, Robert Sparks, and William Grove were particularly instrumental on our behalf.

Other granting agencies have subsequently given their support. These include the U.S. Department of Education's Fund for the Improvement of Post-Secondary Education, with the assistance of Felicia Kaplan and the National Fund for Medical Foundation with the assistance of John Freymann.

The PCC students had a strong enough belief to take a chance on an exciting but untested idea. They worked hard enough to translate that idea into a thriving program. They deserve our endless gratitude, for they have been our greatest teachers. Since PCC is their program, they have reviewed chapter drafts to ensure that this work accurately reflects their experiences. Conventional-track students' voluntary involvement in our education research is also gratefully acknowledged.

With their tireless efforts and ability to share major administrative responsibility, the staff of the Primary Care Curriculum has been a unique asset to the program. Allison Stubbs helped develop the curriculum and organize the case materials in an artistic and lively manner. Lynn Lahren assisted in organizing the research data and in conducting student interviews and observations as well as in data analysis. Kathy Benshoof coordinated data collection and data management. Elizabeth Baca and Kathy Sanchez assumed major managerial functions for the program with the assistance of Troylyn Sisneros, Teresa Mondragon, and Carol Baca. Bill Anglin did the bulk of expert transcribing of the text of this book.

Biostatistical consultation for this work was provided by Dorothy Pathak and Debbie Harrington. Creative artwork was provided by Leona Abeita, Mike Norviel, and Dennis Clark.

We are especially grateful for the wisdom, guidance, and support, as well as needed criticism, of Dean Leonard Napolitano, Sidney Solomon, and Robert Anderson. PCC profited greatly from a team of faculty discipline representatives who provided a sounding board for ideas and concerns about PCC among the basic and clinical science departments. These faculty included Sei Tokuda, William Wiese, Leslie Smith, Linda McGuffey, Don Britton, William Woodside, James Wallace, Robert Kelley, Joan Koss, Charles Key, and Beulah Woodfin.

PCC's Evaluation Committee enjoyed major contributions from Gaynor Wild and Fred Herzon and our Clinical Skills Committee profited from the dedicated teaching contributions of Ed Bernstein, Craig Vanderwagen, Chris Urbina, and Cecilia Dail. Experimental laboratory sessions for PCC students conducted by Jerry Weiss and Don Priola and computer-based problem development by Leslie Dalton III were also greatly appreciated.

We are grateful to Al Atencio and Meg Gabarina for the vital, supportive services they provided to students and for sharing with us ideas about admissions and support of minority students.

The University of New Mexico Medical Center Library has been a unique and creative resource to PCC thanks in large measure to the work of Erica Love, Lillian Croghan, and Susan Chamberlain. Our patient-simulation program took flight under the guiding wings of Sara Voorhees.

Residents of many communities throughout New Mexico welcomed and cared for PCC students during the community-based portions of their education. Ann Starks helped link the University with the preceptorship sites and the following physicians in New Mexico served as preceptors for three of four student rotations: Richard Kozoll, William Lawless, and Leonard Cain in Cuba, N.M.; Allan Firestone in Bernalillo; Doug Dye in Silver City; Robert Shannon and Joseph Dean in Roswell; Alfredo Vigil in Questa; Fred Kullman in Santa Fe; Larry Schrieber in Taos; Edward Fikany in Ft. Summer; David Elliott, Michael Lopez, Judith Vaughn, and George Bunch in Las Vegas, N.M.; Anthony Martinez and Jeffrey Seltz in Los Lunas; David Rouleau in Capitan; and Charles Lehman in Portales. Robin Tuchler from Albuquerque served as a circuit rider for five years.

Many educators from other medical schools worldwide have shared their information freely with us and given us encouragement. In North America, these include Reed Williams, Howard Barrows, Linda

Distlehorst, and Nu Viet Vu at Southern Illinois University; Ellen Tabak at the University of Colorado; Ron Pust at the University of Arizona; Ralph Berggren at Mercer University in Macon, Georgia; John Verby at the University of Minnesota; Jack Jones and Lynda Farquhar at Michigan State University, and Daniel Mazzuchi at Michigan State's Upper Peninsula Program in Marquette; Vic Neufeld at McMaster University in Hamilton, Ontario, Canada; and Leonard Meiselas from the Sophie Davis School of Biomedical Education in New York City.

In Latin America, these include Dra. Maria Teresa Cortes of the National Autonomous University, Mexico City; Dr. Ramon Villarreal, of Metropolitan University, Xochimilco, Mexico; Dr. Jose de Paula Lopes Pontes, University of Rio De Janeiro, Brazil; Dr. Oscar Bolanos, University de Valle, Colombia; and Dr. Humberto Lopez, School of Medicine, Managua, Nicaragua.

In the Middle East, these include Dr. Zohair Nooman, Suez Canal University, Ismailia, Egypt; Dr. Abdulla Saeed Bahattab, University of Aden, Democratic Republic of Yemen; Dr. N. H. Fisk, Hacettepe University, Ankara, Turkey; Dr. Dan E. Benor, Ben-Gurian University, Beersheba, Israel; and Drs. L. M. Epstein and A. Tamir, Technion Faculty of Medicine, Haifa, Israel.

In Africa, these include Prof. B. Hamad, University of Gezira, Wad Medani, Sudan; Dr. E. H. D. Parry, University of Science and Technology, Kumas, Ghana; Dr. Adeoye Adenizy, University of Ilorin, Unilorin, Nigeria; Dr. O. O. Kale, University of Ibadan, Ibadan, Nigeria; and Dr. Isabel Gomes, University Eduardo, Maputo, Mozambique.

In Europe, these include Dr. Carlos Belmonte, University of Alicante, Spain; Prof. J. M. Greep, University of Limburg, Maastricht, Netherlands; Prof. Per Bjurulf, Linkoping University, Sweden; Prof. D. A. S. Beritic-Stahuljak, University of Zagreb, Yugoslavia; Prof. J. B. L. Howell, University of Southampton, Great Britain.

And in Australasia, these include Drs. Graham Feletti and Charles Engel, University of Newcastle, New South Wales, Australia; Prof. M. S. Trastotenojo, Diponegoro University, Semarang University, Indonesia; Dr. Florentino Herrera, Jr., University of the Philippines, Manila; Dr. M. Saidi Hashim Tahir, University Sains Malaysia, Panang; Dr. Vanchai Vatanasapt, Khon Kaen University, Thailand; and Prof. Gopal Archaraya, Tribhuven University, Katmandu, Nepal.

I am grateful to my parents for instilling into me an orientation toward other people's needs and the need for social change.

My brother Marshall Kaufman's superb editing and side-splitting humor were of inestimable value in bringing clarity of thought and

Introduction

"A medical student faints at the sight of blood.
- *Would you expect his pulse to be fast or slow?*
- *What underlying mechanism caused his fainting?"*

This is the kind of problem that first-year medical students in our program are asked to investigate, while their counterparts in traditional medical curricula are trying to memorize the names of all the holes in the skull.

As evidenced in the above example, our program centers on problem-based learning rather than rote memory. This book tells how our program was conceived, how it was implemented, how it is proceeding, what the results have been so far, and what we foresee for the future.

Our program has been instituted at our school, the University of New Mexico (Kaufman et al., 1982). The curriculum runs simultaneously with, but is academically separate from, the traditional curriculum in the first two years and is known as the Primary Care Curriculum, or PCC. In the second two years, students in both tracks work together in clinical clerkships. PCC has two main goals. The first is to graduate physicians who will better address community health needs. The second is to engender self-motivated, lifelong learning skills among its students. These goals have drawn increasing attention internationally among medical educators. One can now find a substantial literature on program design and educational methods addressing these two emerging concerns in medical education. But there is a dearth of material actually recounting and analyzing experiences of those attempting to implement such programs.

As to the first goal, geographic and specialty maldistribution of health care providers remains a major problem. Solutions have been offered by state and federal governments, organized medicine, and universities. But most efforts at influencing career and location of young physicians are made late in their training and do not have the desired effect. The federal government has attempted to attract young physicians to rural communities by establishing the National Health Service Corps, and by supporting programs that fund primary care residency positions. These efforts have resulted in variable success, but they now face ominous budgetary reductions. Less emphasis has been placed on the total pattern of medical education itself, a fact which may underlie much of the current maldistribution.

What of the second goal? Can medical schools better prepare their students to become problem-solvers and self-directed, lifelong learners? Teaching what is currently known does not ensure that the students will learn what will be important in the future. The provision of real patient problems as the core of the curriculum gives the medical student a natural learning stimulus. The subject matter is relevant, and the student exercises reasoning ability while gaining new factual knowledge. It is through this method of teaching that we hope to ensure lifelong learning. The student will become accustomed to learning from the problems presented by patients for whom he cares. But such educational innovations tamper with the age-old separation between the basic and clinical sciences, with departmental control of the curriculum, and with the traditional timing of clinical experiences. The innovators must confront the territorial protectiveness of academic departments within the larger institution.

Major changes in medical education can develop more easily in new medical schools. Illustrative examples of problem-based or community-oriented educational innovations exist at new schools such as the University of Limburg at Maastricht (Bouhuijs et al., 1978), McMaster University Medical School in Ontario (Neufeld & Barrows, 1974), Newcastle in New South Wales (Clarke, 1977), and the Biomedical Education Program at City College in New York (Geiger, 1980). Newly created medical schools can attract faculty members who already believe in the new philosophy, thus reducing the intense political infighting that occurs when planners in an established curriculum attempt major structural change.

However, the economic situation—both current and predicted—is causing a rapid decline of new medical school development in the United States. The vast majority of medical schools in the United States and abroad are traditional. Therefore, major curricular innovations will have to arise within establishments in which those who are seeking such changes will inevitably run a collision course with faculty and administrators with strong vested interests and departmental prerogatives.

PCC has completed a half decade of program implementation. Its planners have come to realize that issues concerning program design and educational theory occupy a lesser portion of their time than originally expected. Of far greater importance to survival of the program has been the ability of innovators to frame new concepts in ways that build bridges with traditionally minded faculty rather than isolate the program from them. Further, the ability to assess the political climate, both within and outside the medical school, and to channel program efforts toward achievable goals is of critical importance if the innovation is to survive.

One researcher's laboratory experiment or one department's educational innovation can proceed without intense scrutiny or need for approval from other departments. But this is not the case for those attempting broad educational reforms that cut across all basic and clinical science disciplines. Although many faculty have embraced PCC's methods, others have seen PCC as a threat to their basic beliefs about medical education. Reaction by faculty critics has ranged from helpful suggestions to coolness to outright hostility. PCC faculty have often felt worn down by the criticism, sensed a futility in trying to make inroads in traditional belief systems, and longed for refuge in less controversial endeavors.

What is it, though, that sustained the interest of the innovators? What sustained them in the face of external criticism, paucity of formal rewards, and, for some, risk to reputation and promotion? Why do they now continue to give so much time to the new program, when the bulk of inspirational planning has long been completed? The reason most PCC faculty and staff would offer is the intense personal reward of observing the effect of the experimental program on its students. The students' enthusiasm for learning, and the students' personal investment in working diligently to make their program better, offer faculty and staff a "natural high." In this setting in which students, faculty, and staff function as colleagues, there emerges a special, intimate relationship among participants, encouraging a feeling of "family." This is at once rare in medical school, appropriate for a graduate program in the helping professions, and magnetic in its bonding of participants to the common effort, even in the face of adversity.

Over the years, PCC faculty and staff have been serving as educational consultants to faculty from many other medical schools that are seeking similar curricular change. Thus, the need for a document that would go beyond theory and clearly lay out practical steps in implementing a problem-based curriculum has become apparent.

This book, therefore, explores in depth one program, PCC, because its development, successes, and failures are known intimately by the authors. However, the New Mexico program is but one of many problem-based curricular innovations that have emerged worldwide in recent years. It is thus important to compare PCC with other programs to determine what elements in the implementation of problem-based learning are universal, and what elements are unique to PCC. Consequently, each chapter illustrates various approaches to its topic with examples from select programs.

After the first chapter on the inception of PCC and other key programs, each chapter will begin with a statement of the specific goals toward which a problem-based learning curriculum should strive. The PCC experience, in attempting to achieve these objectives, will then be presented with an analysis of successes and failures and a summary of the main points learned over the years. A sampling of experiences of other medical schools experimenting with problem-based learning will then be reviewed.

By detailing the development and early results of the program at the University of New Mexico, and by reviewing the experiences of other medical schools engaged in experiments in problem-based learning, we hope to illustrate the many avenues and barriers to institutional change. We feel that readers will profit from a "front-line" account of this experience.

In the process of changing our curriculum, far more time than planned was spent in the trench warfare of institutional politics, and less in the more lofty intellectual pursuits concerning program design and evaluation. But should one expect anything different? Such curriculum innovations find a more receptive audience among consumers, educational theorists, practicing physicians, and legislators. But those most intimately involved in medical education are medical school faculty members who, by training and professional interest, are often most distant from the eventual professional lives of the students they educate. Bridging this gap between education and practice is an arduous, but very rewarding task.

It is important that our false assumptions and errors of judgment, as well as our successes, be clearly described. The power of problem-based learning to release the creative energy of students and faculty is extraordinary. But while it is inherently attractive as a concept, its realization can be elusive if curriculum innovators fail to assess accurately their institution's climate for change. For the idea to take root, it must be sampled by a broad representation of faculty. For the idea to flourish, planners of innovation must be willing to share its ownership and be open to criticism and change.

References

Bouhuijs, P. A. S., Schmidt, H. G., Snow, R. E., & Wignen, W. H. F. W. (1978). The Rijksuniversitet Limburg, Maastricht, Netherlands: Development of medical education. *Public Health Papers, 70,* 133–151, Geneva: WHO.

Clarke, R. M. (1977). The new medical school at Newcastle, New South Wales. *The Lancet, 1,* 434–435.

Geiger, J. H. (1980). Sophie Davis School of Biomedical Education at City College of New York prepares primary care physicians for practice in underserved inner-city areas. *Public Health Reports, 95,* 32–37.

Kaufman, A., Klepper, D., Obenshain, S. S., Voorhees, J. D., Galey, W., Duban, S., Moore-West, M., Jackson, R., Bennett, M., & Waterman, R. (1982). Undergraduate medical education for rural primary care: A case study in New Mexico. *Southern Medical Journal, 75,* 1110–1117.

Neufeld, V. R., & Barrows, H. S. (1974). The McMaster philosophy: An approach to medical education. *Journal of Medical Education, 49,* 1040–50.

CHAPTER 1

Origins

ARTHUR KAUFMAN AND S. SCOTT OBENSHAIN

The likelihood of change is enhanced when there is a crisis in the environment, when people have a shared interest in change, when there is a power imbalance in the environment, when the environment has experienced structural changes, and finally, when it is consistent with the zeitgeist or spirit of the times. (Levine, 1980, p. 6)

The authors came to New Mexico to be part of a medical school that was responsive to community health needs. In this relatively poor, tricultural state, there were palpable community health issues which drew the interest and imagination of many at the medical center.

Yet the curriculum at the medical school bore no particular relationship to the problems of New Mexico.

Too often students perceived their teachers as adversaries rather than colleagues.

"I listen to their lectures and take their tests in a large, anonymous lecture hall. But I don't get close to many of the faculty. I feel like I'm always on trial, jumping through their hoops, not yet worthy of their trust."

Too often students viewed their coursework as more of a hurdle than an educational adventure.

"I don't see the point of all this material they're throwing at us. They don't connect it with patients or any real problems. But I'm not going to make waves. I'm just going to get through."

And too often the idealism of students bent on serving their fellow man was dampened by the overly demanding schedule on campus of classroom and homework.

> *"I wanted to be more human and not lose touch with my friends. I wanted to continue running my church youth program and maybe teach the kids about first aid and disease prevention. But look what I've become—a drone. I sit in one class after another. I study all evening. I've had to drop my church work and worry that my friends will drift off."*

Since their arrival at the medical school, Kaufman and Obenshain have sought a new direction—to create a learning environment for students based on the needs of the state and to develop a curriculum that capitalized on students' enthusiasm to learn and dedication to service.

Experimenting with the Family and Community Medical Curriculum

Dr. Art Kaufman, a family physician and internist, was an Assistant Professor, who, when he arrived at the Department of Family and Community Medicine, had been assigned the task of starting its undergraduate program. The first course he tried was entitled "Introduction to Family and Community Medicine" for first-year students. It consisted of a two-hour lecture, one afternoon a week. Each week a different faculty member would lecture, covering a topic in his particular area of expertise. Kaufman had watched in anguish as the course received yawns and underwhelming reviews from the class. Many of the faculty who taught in the course were viewed as excellent attending physicians in the hospital, but they were perceived as inept teachers in the lecture hall. The negative reaction from the students was a blow to the Department and, for Kaufman, a painful déjà vu experience. A decade before as a medical student, he had led a student rebellion against what he felt to be inept teaching in a similar course in his own medical school. Now he was getting the same criticisms he once gave. Humbled, he sought alternatives.

Kaufman reflected upon two of his important previous learning experiences—one in the Indian Health Service; the other, residency. After internship, and prior to residency, Kaufman spent two years in rural communities in South Dakota and New Mexico working with health teams in the Indian Health Service. In these settings, health care problems of individuals clearly reflected the social, political, and economic problems of the community from which the individuals came.

Adequate preparation for providing care appeared to require as much knowledge of cultural anthropology, epidemiology, and health economics, as it did of biochemistry and physiology. His education had not prepared Kaufman for this demand.

Before joining the New Mexico faculty, Kaufman completed a residency in internal medicine. He had been struck by the role of the ward team as a powerful stimulus for learning. Each team consisted of a small group of residents, interns, and medical students who lived and worked together, shared frustrations, provided social support, and stimulated one another's learning. He recalled how joyful and purposeful this team-learning seemed, compared with his earlier feelings of alienation while sitting as a medical student in the rear of a dimly lit, cavernous lecture hall. He recalled the terror of listening to a biochemist exhort the class to memorize the lecture material under the threat, "If you don't know this you'll be a killer after you graduate."

These two experiences, the Indian Health Service and residency, had been the most exciting, intense periods of learning in his life. All learning was experiential, in context, and stimulated by real patient and community problems. Further, it was shared and broadened by small groups of fellow health workers. Why must education in medical school, especially in the preclinical years, be so remote from that excitement? Must students remain passive and anonymous in a classroom, and function in relative isolation from each other? Must they be driven more by fear of an examination than by love of learning? Must their scientific learning be vicarious through texts and lectures rather than through the personal experience of grappling with a scientific problem? Was such traditional, sheltered, lecture-hall learning a necessary antecedent to the later clinical experiences?

Rebounding from the failure of that first course he had organized, Kaufman now guided his faculty's teaching efforts in a radically different direction. The string of weekly lectures was converted into a solid week course for all students. There were no lectures. There was no passive student learning. The class was divided into small groups, and the faculty led the groups in discussions of clinical problems (Chapter 6). Basic and clinical science issues were both brought into the discussions. Instruction on physical examination skills was included in the sessions, and each student attended a community-health-related facility such as Alcoholics Anonymous during one of the evenings. The students' enthusiasm for the course was overwhelming. They regarded this participatory, student-centered method of learning as one of the high points of their curriculum.

The upshot was a student demand for more instruction on physical examination and more small-group and community learning experiences. The Department responded with a brief course on more advanced clinical-skills training. It then set up a series of community-based clinical electives, expanding the contact time between faculty and students (Voorhees et al., 1977). Although the students were excited by these new methods, and could better appreciate the relationship between clinical and basic sciences, the didactic onslaught of the concurrent, traditional courses neutralized the effect of much of the newer innovations. In light of his department's success with this new format of education, Kaufman wondered whether the entire preclinical medical curriculum could be organized in this fashion.

The Office of Undergraduate Medical Education

Scott Obenshain, a pediatrician, had been Assistant Dean of Undergraduate Medical Education for the Medical School for two of the five years he had been at the institution. His background had been in academia, having done research in metabolism. After three years as Director of the Pediatric Clinic, his time was now spent in meeting with faculty committees, developing student-evaluation norms, deciding which students would pass and fail, and advising students who were in serious academic and/or personal difficulty. Many students adjusted poorly to medical school and seemed isolated. Heading an Office of Education rather than a Department of Education, his contacts were many but his power was limited. Power resided within each Department, and coordinating their efforts into a new direction in education seemed an elusive goal. The focus of committee meetings often had more to do with competing requests over departmental teaching hours than with educational philosophy. Obenshain was frustrated, and he sensed that much of the student stress so evident in his office was related to curriculum design and methods of instruction. These, at times, pitted teacher and student against each other, rather than bringing them together in an optimal learning environment.

Though the medical school was only ten years old, much of its early energy was fading. A number of the chairmen with whom Obenshain dealt had been present from the early days of the school—when the curriculum was more innovative, when classes were small, and when student–faculty relations were close. The school had initially incorporated the innovative organ-system approach from Western Reserve instead of traditional discipline courses for most of the preclinical courses. But by now some of the faculty's enthusiasm for educational innovation had dampened. They complained that they did not receive proper recognition for their teaching efforts by their chairmen, for their efforts were now melded with those of faculty from many other departments. Thus, pressure was growing to return to traditional, departmental course teaching. Obenshain saw that a rebirth of enthusiasm for innovation was needed. How could he generate the spark that would ignite interest in change?

One of the most creative educational endeavors with which Obenshain had been associated was the development of an experiment headed by Dr. Robert Oseasohn, the Chairman of the school's fledgling Department of Community Medicine. The department trained the first rural family nurse practitioner in the United States. She was to function in a New Mexico site remote from her physician supervisors (Oseasohn et al., 1971). The effort focused upon Estancia, a county seat in a sparsely populated, relatively poor, farming/ranching district located 60 miles from Albuquerque, across the Sandia Mountains. Though the community had built a clinic to attract a physician replacement for its retired general practitioner, a permanent physician could not be found. The community therefore negotiated with the University to develop a demonstration linkage system. A physician would visit the clinic once weekly. But a nurse would be stationed there five days a week and would provide care under telephone backup supervision by physicians at the medical school. A nurse was selected who had strong ties to the community (her husband was a local rancher), and she underwent six months of medical training at the University. Protocols for patient care, simple laboratory tests, and referral were carefully designed. With increased health care skills, a bundle of treatment and referral protocols at her disposal, and a telephone backup system in place, the first rural family nurse practitioner commenced a successful, pioneering career in rural New Mexico. Shortly thereafter, one of the nation's first nurse practitioner training programs began at the University of New Mexico.

The education of that nurse had particular relevance for medical education at the University. Unmet community health needs had created a demand for new educational solutions, and educational innovation had drawn the expertise of the University out into a needy area of the state. Further, the nurse practitioner's expanded training and responsibilities had planted the seeds for new career opportunities in nursing. A number of nursing schools, for example, were now experimenting with entry and exit points in a career-ladder curriculum which led from a nurse's aide to a licensed practical nurse (LPN) to a registered nurse (RN). At each step, the student could exit with a marketable skill. Obenshain lamented at the contrast between the freedom of that model and the constraints inherent in medical education. Medical students could not obtain an interim degree, exit from school temporarily, and market their skill. Obenshain wondered whether medical education could be redesigned to provide more flexibility to provide students with a career-ladder model.

The Community

Kaufman and Obenshain noted other forces in New Mexico that were creating demands for a new direction in medical education. A problem increasingly discussed nationally was the maldistribution of physicians both by geography and by specialty.

New Mexico represented the epitome of the problem. As the fifth largest state geographically, yet with a small population (about 1.3 million people), New Mexico is typical of many Rocky Mountain states that have a concentration of people in a limited number of areas with the remainder spread over vast expanses. Approximately 30 percent of New Mexico's population is concentrated within three central cities that lie within a circle with a radius of 40 miles: Albuquerque, Los Alamos, and Santa Fe. The remaining population of about 900,000 is distributed over more than 120,000 square miles. Access to, and coordination of, medical services outside of the three central cities are often limited and, in some cases, nonexistent.

Specialty maldistribution was another problem, and it was getting worse. Congressional testimony in 1976 indicated that in the prior decade a smaller-than-ever percentage of physicians had entered the primary-care specialties of family practice, general internal medicine, general pediatrics, and obstetrics/gynecology.

Need for primary medical care throughout New Mexico was a particularly acute problem. In 1972, compared to other states, New Mexico ranked *forty-ninth* in primary care physicians per one thousand population.

Consideration for the establishment of a medical school at the University of New Mexico had begun during the twenty-fourth session of the New Mexico State Legislature in 1960. The report of the Medical Education Study Committee of that session states:

> The time has come when New Mexico must make provision for the direct education of its own medical students. . . . A related goal is to increase the supply of physicians to meet health needs of the state. (Bennett, 1975, p. 5)

The medical school was thus established with a long-range objective of meeting the health care needs of New Mexico. The first class of 24 students entered in 1964, and class size gradually increased to a steady 73 students per year. Yet by the early 1970s few medical graduates were subsequently returning to underserved areas of the state. The 1977 legislature made a more pointed request.

> . . . the Legislative Finance Committee urges the medical school to formulate a plan to encourage doctors to practice in rural areas where

— LRC —

there is an inadequate level of available medical care. (New Mexico Congress, 1977)

The concern about maldistribution of medical care in New Mexico had thus become a legislative issue.

Medical education today exists in large, urban, academic medical centers, and it concentrates on providing highly technical subspecialty care. Thus, the predominant role model for today's medical student is the tertiary-care specialist practicing in an urban-based referral hospital. From premedical through postgraduate medical training, the typical academic environment fosters the education of highly specialized physicians who, by training and experience, tend to be comfortable locating near urban, tertiary-care facilities capable of supporting their specialties. It seemed that medical education was addressing the health care needs of urban medical centers. The time was ripe for a dramatic redirection in medical education in New Mexico.

Kaufman and Obenshain decided that they would begin to write a "dream" proposal that would revamp the medical school curriculum. The ultimate development, revision, and implementation of that proposal would carry them through a bittersweet adventure in medical education. Bursts of enthusiasm and creativity would be tempered, rerouted, or squelched as they confronted entrenched interests, economic realities, and changing local and national priorities. While the evolving program was chiseled and molded, it was to adapt ever more closely to the local character and needs of its university and state.

Initial Proposal

Their proposal, with a one-year planning budget request of $42,000, was entitled "Pilot Project for Development of a Primary Care Medical School Track Beginning with Physician Assistant Training," and contained the following five goals:

1. To educate highly qualified primary care providers who will work in underserved areas.
2. To provide an educational program that fosters interest in and teaches skills for the delivery of primary health care.
3. To revise the teaching of clinical and basic sciences in medical school so that their interrelationship is better appreciated by the medical student.
4. To revise the teaching of basic sciences in medical school so that it is more clinically relevant, better appreciated by the student, and less of a duplication of college coursework.

5. To enable medical students to provide needed community health care during their medical education.

The Program consisted of three phases culminating in an M.D. degree:

Phase I. Students will enter a physician's assistant (PA) training program lasting approximately two years. The first year will entail didactic and clinical training in Albuquerque. The students will then spend the major portion of their second year as PA preceptees throughout New Mexico in areas of medical need.

Phase II. Students will return to the medical center for a more advanced study of science basic to medicine. This phase will build upon the science basic to PA training, the independent study, and clinical experience of Phase I.

Phase III. The final phase will consist of advanced clinical clerkships, emphasizing increasing patient responsibility.

The immediate faculty reaction to this novel proposal was generally favorable. The more sober criticisms were not to come until later.

Seeking Funding

There ensued a year-long effort to generate funding for the project. In light of the rural, primary care orientation of the proposal, Kaufman consulted with one of his mentors, Dr. Kurt Deuschle, "Father of Community Medicine," and Chairman of the Department of Community Medicine at Mt. Sinai School of Medicine in New York City. Deuschle's first choice of a funding source was the W.K. Kellogg Foundation, distinguished, he felt, by a good track record in educational innovation. He was more skeptical about funding opportunities at The Robert Wood Johnson Foundation and the Commonwealth Fund, both of which Kaufman hoped to visit while traveling in the East. Kaufman made appointments with Johnson and Commonwealth nonetheless. Neither would fund the proposal, and the comment of one officer at Commonwealth was disheartening. Innovations of the magnitude we were proposing, he said, would be less appealing to a foundation because it was coming from a small school in a rural state like New Mexico, rather than coming from a more prestigious, private, trend-setting institution like Yale, Stanford, or Rochester. The proposal was rejected.

Dismayed, Kaufman returned to New Mexico and sent the proposal to the last hope, Kellogg. Kellogg responded by saying that they did not fund planning grants. Prospects now looked dismal, and many months passed with hope for the proposal waning. But in the spring of 1976 there was an almost magical occurrence. Kaufman was driving with his wife and daughter from Albuquerque to New York on vacation. While driving through Chicago, Kaufman decided, on a lark, to call the W.K. Kellogg Foundation in Battle Creek, Michigan, and ask if he could discuss the proposal with an officer at the Foundation. The Foundation's response was cordial, and an interview was arranged for two days later.

At Kellogg, Mr. Andrew Patullo, Vice President of the Foundation, invited Kaufman to lunch. Sunk in the dining room's high-backed leather chairs, the two explored the grant request. Patullo agreed that the New Mexico project was addressing one of Kellog's funding priorities, and he felt that they could make an exception and fund the planning grant, with the understanding that Kellogg would receive first consideration on the full program grant after the planning year. Kaufman floated out of the restaurant.

The planning grant was officially approved some months later when Dr. Robert Sparks, former Vice President for Health Sciences at the University of Nebraska, assumed the role of Medical Director of the Kellogg Foundation. Funding for planning started in November 1976.

The Barrows Connection

In early January 1977, Obenshain learned that one of the medical educators from McMaster University in Canada, Dr. Howard Barrows, was arriving in Albuquerque to review a teaching grant. Barrows had been instrumental in developing the innovative, problem-based curriculum at McMaster. It was hoped that he would offer guidance in developing ideas for the full program proposal. The only available time he would have was 10:00 P.M. at the airport just before his departure. Obenshain, Kaufman, and Dr. Dayton Voorhees, a new faculty member in Family and Community Medicine who was later to develop the entire rural phase of the program, met with Barrows in an airport cafe. The meeting had an electrifying effect on the New Mexico group, as Barrows spoke of the simplicity of the concept of problem-based learning and of its research-based rationale. Barrows pointed out that New Mexico's curricular successes and failures and the students' anguish and joy in medical school had an almost "scientific" explanation. He noted that students, unbridled, possessed an almost boundless energy and capacity to learn. And in a student-centered, problem-based curriculum, the nature of faculty–student relationships would change, the students' energy would be released, and the faculty would earn a far richer reward for the control they relinquished. His clear thinking about problem-based learning was anchored to sound educational research findings. Barrows was later to publish a signal work in the field with his colleague, Robyn Tamblyn, *Problem-Based Learning, An Approach to Medical Education* (Barrows & Tamblyn, 1980).

Though the New Mexico program was later to develop in a direction somewhat different from McMaster's, the structure and clarity Barrows offered during the planning period was invaluable in helping the New Mexico program to articulate its goals and to convert ideas into action.

Advice and Approval

The 1977 planning year saw a flurry of conferences with medical school faculty; meetings with various external consultants; and visits to key experimental medical programs nationally, including Michigan State, McMaster, City College of New York, Duke, Bowman-Gray, and the University of Illinois at Urbana. Political groundwork was laid at home by explaining the proposal to such groups as the Committee of Chairmen, the Curriculum Committee, the Admissions Committees, and the Liaison Committee, which operated between the medical school and the State Medical Society. A faculty advisory committee was established, comprised of representatives from various departments external to the planning group. This committee, in various forms, operated over the ensuing five years and served the critical functions of reflecting general faculty interests and concerns, and of identifying the program areas that needed changes. At this time the program's first name was decided upon: Curriculum for Primary Care (CPC), a play on the traditional CPC or clinical-pathologic conference.

A Warning from the Medical School Accreditors

In mid-April, Kaufman flew to Chicago to meet with representatives of both the American Medical Association and the Association of American Medical Colleges Liaison Committee on Medical Education (LCME), the medical school accrediting body, for approval in concept of the initial CPC plan. The AAMC had two pertinent accrediting groups—one for physician's assistant (PA) programs, and one for medical school programs. Kaufman was disappointed by both groups. The representative for PA programs said that the portion of the CPC plan requesting Physician's Assistant accreditation for students completing their second year was, politically, an untimely request. PA program organizers, he said, were seeking to build an esprit de corps among graduates, whom they hoped would see themselves in terminal careers and not as intermediaries to be siphoned off into medical school. The

CPC plan merely raised the spectre of PA certification becoming a stepping stone toward an M.D. degree. The request was therefore unacceptable.

The medical school accrediting group was quite blunt. While medical schools themselves had the responsibility of determining their own education course, the notion of a career ladder built on PA certification was unacceptable to that accrediting body, for it would "bastardize medical *education* by incorporating within it physician assistant *training*."

It was clear that to force this issue might beach the entire effort in an attempt to preserve one project component. The career-ladder concept was thus removed from the final proposal. This was the first of many compromises made in order for the program to survive, and was, in retrospect, an important experience in perspective and priorities. But although the Chicago meetings did lead to removal of PA accreditation as a mid-curricular end-point, they did not alter the basic plan of education.

Approval by Faculty, Approval by Kellogg

During the spring and summer of 1977, Barrows and Tamblyn conducted a workshop on problem-based learning for UNM faculty; there was a series of visits to McMaster to refine the proposal further and to answer lingering questions about problem-based methods; and meetings between CPC planners and other faculty increased. At one planning meeting, Dr. Sidney Solomon, Chairman of Physiology, expressed a concern about the increasing time demands on department representatives helping to plan for CPC. He convinced CPC planners that continued meeting of these demands might depend upon a clear vote of support for the new proposed program by the faculty as a whole. Obenshain and Kaufman therefore distributed a six-page update on the CPC plan to all faculty. The document addressed many of the faculty concerns heard during the planning period. Many faculty feared growing demands on their teaching responsibilities without additional reward or compensation. Some faculty worried that once the new track commenced it would be irreversible. Others worried that the educational standards of the school might be compromised—that a system that was working fairly well in providing a quality education was being challenged unjustly, and that a track stressing primary care would surely serve as a back door to medical school for weaker students.

Dean Leonard Napolitano placed the subject of CPC on the agenda of the September 1, 1977, quarterly general faculty meeting. One of the largest faculty turnouts unanimously approved the proposal by voice vote. The years of careful planning, and the seeking of broad support and consensus, were reaping their rewards—another milestone in the development of CPC had been reached. Dean Napolitano conveyed the enthusiastic support of the faculty to Dr. Robert Sparks at Kellogg, and a final, 214-page grant request for $4.4 million over a 5½-year period was submitted. The CPC planning group's hopes for funding were high.

Kellogg approved the grant in May 1978, but for only $680,000 over a three-year period. CPC planners were shattered. The original proposed budget had been "fat" with funds to each department to "bring them on board." Because of Kaufman's belief in Kellogg's enthusiasm for the project, and because of the faculty's overwhelming support, it was assumed that the proposal would be approved for the full amount. There had been no consideration of how to manage the program on less. A flurry of meetings ensued in which faculty and staff debated whether the program should begin at all. In retrospect, the concern seems almost comical in light of how well the program did function. But at the time, the future looked uncertain.

When planners finally agreed to proceed within the scaled-down budget, the nature of activity changed. What had seemed to be endless theoretical planning meetings now became hard-nosed, task-oriented meetings in which tangible products, such as case problems and evaluation materials, were developed.

It was decided to accept a small class of ten students the first year. They were arriving shortly. Department efforts and concerns sharpened. Each department developed its own posture vis-à-vis CPC. One department saw teaching as a faculty function and declared incentive money to be unnecessary for their participation. But another requested $5,000 to support a graduate student. A third begrudgingly said they would work with CPC though they had little faith in its underlying philosophy of education.

The prior unanimous approval given to CPC belied the serious and growing doubts harbored by many about the program. Those doubts would emerge both subtly and in full force as CPC was transformed from a theoretical plan—an idea nurtured by a few faculty—to a highly visible educational track whose ideas were aggressively promoted by its founders and students.

And Then, Name Changes

During 1979, as program planners anxiously awaited student applications and selection for the first CPC class, a curious set of external events led to two name changes for the fledgling educational track. Before the first class arrived, the letters "CPC" were not "household" initials around the medical school. When a new Child Psychiatric Center was dedicated on campus in 1978 "CPC" became popularized for that new facility. The Curriculum for Primary Care therefore sought a new designation, and settled on Curriculum for Rural Primary Care, "RPC" for short. However, this enjoyed a rather brief life, because representatives from smaller New Mexico communities complained that the term "rural," when employed by a city dweller, is often perceived as demeaning—implying "backward" or "bumpkin." One physician defined "rural" as the town down the road that had one fewer doctor than the one in which you were raised. Consequently, the name changed, for the last time, to "Primary Care Curriculum" or "PCC." This final name expressed the program's orientation without offending part of its constituency.

Developing Goals

Before the first class of students arrived, and as the curriculum was being assembled, it became evident that it was quite important that the goals of the program be very clearly stated. This would not only be a guide for both the students and the faculty, but it would also serve as a basis for evaluating the results of the program. We settled upon nine goals, as stated in the following boxes.

---

1. *Scientific Reasoning.* The student will be able to approach clinical problems with appropriate scientific reasoning (identifying and rank ordering problems, generating and testing broad hypotheses), while integrating information from the basic and clinical science disciplines. The student will be able to function effectively in an environment of ambiguity and uncertainty.

2. *Scientific Content.* The student will attain a working knowledge of the basic and clinical sciences and will be able to describe pertinent abnormal physical or behavioral processes and their interrelationships in all the patient's identified problems. The student should be able to describe these events in appropriate pathophysiological, psychological, or sociological terms, listing the facts that support the processes identified. If the student feels that several possibilities exist on the basis of the data available, they should be listed in order of importance (likelihood, urgency, etc.).

3. *Research Assessment Skills.* When studying a medically related report (journal, monograph, paper, presentation, abstract, etc.), the student will be able to assess critically the question being posed and its significance; the appropriateness and limitations of the methods being used; the consistencies and significance of the data and whether the conclusions are consistent with the data; the remaining unanswered questions; and the relevance of the information to current problems.

(continued)

(*continued*)

4. *Resource Utilization.*   When faced with medical problems requiring further expertise for proper diagnosis or management, the student will be able to identify and utilize efficiently an appropriate quantity and quality of resources including texts, journal articles, library and community resources, and faculty.

5. *Lifelong Learning.*   The student will continue to demonstrate a high level of motivation in the pursuit of the science basic to medicine. She or he will demonstrate the ability to utilize interaction with patient problems as a stimulus for self-directed study.

6. *Collection and Presentation of Data.*   The student will be able to collect adequate data from the patient, using the appropriate range of interview and examination skills. The student will be able to organize the information into a concise, problem-oriented document, and succinctly present the problem and its analysis orally.

7. *Interpersonal Skills.*   The student will be able to demonstrate the interpersonal skills and cultural awareness necessary to facilitate patient communication, patient understanding of her or his problem(s), and proposed management and patient comfort. The student will be able to demonstrate insightful and constructive self and peer criticism. The student will demonstrate the ability to build a team relationship with other students and health professionals, appropriately identifying and utilizing their input in problem assessment and management.

8. *Community and Family Health.*   The student will be able to demonstrate an ability to describe the impact of the health problem on the patient, the patient's family, and the community. The student will be able to identify family relationships, and factors in the community and environment, which might have influenced positively or negatively the identified health problems. The student will be able to assess the interaction between the patient and the community in terms of health prevention and maintenance.

9. *Cost Containment.*   The student will be able to indicate the cost of proposed treatment and management and demonstrate an understanding of the mechanisms whereby patients are able to pay for health care services.

What We Have Learned

1. *It is important to create goals which will describe the behaviors that students will exhibit upon graduation and in later practice.*   This will give coherence to the problem-based program plan, it will guide the selection of students, and it will help in the selection of the clinical curriculum topics. It will assist in the selection of evaluation techniques and in the setting of priorities for applications for supporting funds.

2. *Goals should be selected which reflect the unique values of the proposed program.* Goals should reflect the particular needs and values of the institution and its community. These aspects will determine, for example, the relative balance between classroom, laboratory, hospital, and community learning experiences, and the degree of student responsibility for learning.

3. *It is important to identify forces promoting and resisting the program.* In early program planning, energy must be channeled into creative development of ideas and action. Precious time and energy can be diverted from productive work into wasteful confrontations with faculty who are resistant to the proposed change. Building a support group identity is critically important in this early stage.

4. *The base of support for the new program should be broadened early.* To prevent a "we" versus "them" attitude among faculty, incorporate the ideas of as large a representative group as possible in the planning stages. A broad base of support is needed in the early, more fragile phases of development.

5. *It is important to seek areas of agreement with conventionally minded faculty.* Acknowledge curricular elements in conventional education which are of agreed value, and build a case for needed change from shared concerns with conventional faculty. Early polarization of faculty diminishes the likelihood of a later cooperative effort.

References

Barrows, H. S., & Tamblyn R. M. (1980). *Problem based learning, an approach to medical education.* New York: Springer Publishing Company.

Bennett, M. (1975, December). Medical manpower in New Mexico. *New Mexico Business,* pp. 3–10.

Levine, A. (1980). *Why innovation fails.* Albany: State University of New York Press.

New Mexico Congress. (1977). Legislative Finance Committee. Budget Analysis—Selected State Agencies, 33 leg., 1st Session, p. 40.

Oseasohn, R., Mortimer, E. A., Geil, C. C., Eberle, B. S., Pressmen, A. E., & Quenck, N. L. (1971). Rural medical care: physician's assistant linked to an urban medical center. *JAMA, 218,* 1417–1419.

Voorhees, J. D., Kaufman, A., Heffron, W., Jackson, R., DiVasto, P., Wiese, W., & Daitz, B. (1977). Teaching pre-clinical medical students in a clinical setting. *Journal of Family Practice, 5,* 464–465.

CHAPTER 2

Curriculum: Problems to Stimulate Learning

ROBERT E. WATERMAN AND COOLEY BUTLER

"Absolutely perfect session! Group worked well, all contributed productively. Went from discussion of how to read chest X-rays, to gross anatomy of the lung and pleura, to histology of pulmonary capillary beds, to mechanics of respiration, to fluid dynamics in different capillary beds, to sequence of events occurring after left AV valve stenosis, to effect of decreased pH on respiratory control centers, and were getting to biochemical issues when we had to stop because of another scheduled event. Had a short evaluation. Everyone excited by the morning. Victor less anxious, Peggy did outstanding job at board with drawings and explanations." (PCC tutor's field notes—First-year tutorial)

Goals of a Curriculum in Problem-Based Learning

1. The curriculum should stimulate the student's self-directed learning. Problems should be developed which introduce students to core scientific concepts deemed appropriate for that phase of study.

2. Students should encounter problems in the manner in which a physician would.
3. The curriculum should challenge the student to select information efficiently from a variety of sources.
4. The curriculum should challenge the student to integrate information from a broad range of scientific disciplines.
5. Problems should challenge the student to exercise and develop clinical reasoning.
6. Problems should facilitate students' increasing comfort in the face of clinical uncertainty.

Introduction

We are entering the Information Age (Naisbitt, 1982). Over 6,000 scientific articles are written each day, and much of that information will soon become obsolete. It is no longer sufficient to teach medical students today's "state-of-the-art" science. The physician of the future must learn how to learn, how to select and integrate appropriate information to diagnose and manage their patients' problems in the best possible manner.

It is troubling, then, to note the disparity between how physicians will have to learn in the future and how medical students are taught today. Large lecture-hall learning is the predominant form of instruction in the preclinical years. Students are passive learners and receive answers to questions they may not have asked. A British study of student concentration during lectures showed an almost universal peak at 10 to 15 minutes with a steady decline thereafter (Stuart & Rutherford, 1978). The curriculum is lock-stepped for the efficiency of the teacher more than the learner. Rogers appeared shaken after his brush with contemporary preclinical medical education and characterized the attempt to learn basic sciences in the current, overcrowded lecture schedule as "like trying to drink water from a fire hose" (Rogers, 1982). He recommended cutting the curriculum by 40 percent, simply to give students time to breathe, think, and digest what is presented. This sentiment is widespread, and a number of medical schools have provided unscheduled time for their students during the week.

Problem-based learning allows individualization of instruction, helping students to focus on issues they deem relevant. By allowing students to take some control over the direction, speed, and depth of their study, frustration is diminished and the learning environment is more conducive to creativity and enthusiasm. Two questions facing those who wish to implement changes in medical education are (1) How can a problem-based curriculum be introduced into medical school? (2) How can it evolve and adapt in a manner acceptable to the institution? The introduction of such a clinically oriented, problem-based, student-centered curriculum may not be well accepted by conventional faculty accustomed to controlling the content and organization of student learning. If such faculty do not value the process of learning at least as much as its content, then a strong negative reaction will emerge. George Miller's observation of Buffalo's experiment in tutorial learning in the 1950s underscores this point.

> [Reaction] was especially intense among those who believed that there was barely enough time during the first year to deal effectively with the most basic preclinical sciences, and that such seductive entertainment (i.e., tutorial group meetings) simply distracted students from more important academic tasks. (Miller, 1980)

New Mexico Program

Overview of PCC Curriculum

Two of the basic principles adopted by the small number of individuals who planned the initial PCC curriculum were:

1. Students should encounter a balance of patient care settings; urban and rural, primary and tertiary care.
2. The method of learning should instill in students an active, lifelong learning capability.

While these concepts remain as the basic foundation of the curriculum, the means to accomplish them have undergone significant change. The four-year PCC curriculum is divided into three major phases, as illustrated in Figure 2.1. The first phase, which occupies the first year, is subdivided into two parts—Phases IA and IB. The second year is designated Phase II; the third and fourth years are combined as Phase III.

Curriculum development has focused primarily upon the first two years of the medical school, since Phase III is comprised of traditional hospital clerkships, and is, by nature, already "problem-based" and clinically oriented. Innovations in these latter years are just now being formulated.

Phase IA: Clinical Problem-Based Tutorials. This phase occupies the first six months of medical school. During this time, students work in tutorial groups of five students and one faculty facilitator. The

Figure 2.1. Four-year schedule of primary care curriculum.

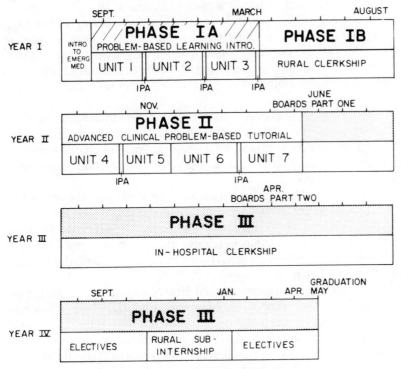

group meets for a half-day session three times a week. Phase IA is divided into three units, which last approximately eight weeks each. The clinical problems encountered by students during Phase IA are designed to introduce techniques of problem-based learning and to provide a survey of the major concepts in each of the basic science disciplines.

Tutorials also emphasize interpersonal and group skills (Chapter 3). Students learn to work in a team and to listen critically. Self and peer evaluation is an important aspect of the tutorial experience. Students can compare their own performance with that of their peers and practice the skills required to make clear and concise presentations. The tutorial also provides an opportunity for students to recognize and discuss their emotional reactions to various issues such as death, sexuality, and medical ethics.

During the first 15 weeks of Phase IA, the students also participate in a problem-based, clinical skills session one morning per week (Chapter 5). Here they learn the skills and scientific basis of a routine history and physical examination. They will need these abilities when they enter the second part of the freshman year, Phase IB.

A typical weekly schedule for PCC students during Phase IA is shown in Figure 2.2. A large part of the students' time is spent in independent study, pursuing topics and learning issues either derived from tutorial sessions or self-generated. Some time is also spent interacting with faculty members who act as important resources for learning.

By the end of Phase IA, students have begun to develop the skills necessary to interact with patients. They are becoming more comfortable with the anatomical and physiological basis of the physical examination, and they are able to identify relevant learning issues from patient interactions.

Phase IB. During the remaining four to six months of the first year, students are required to participate in a preceptorship located in a medically underserved area, usually at a site distant from the main campus. The students, often in teams, live in a rural community and work with a physician preceptor. This portion of the curriculum is fully described in Chapter 7.

Phase II. The students spend their second year back at the School of Medicine in an advanced, problem-based tutorial phase. They now meet twice weekly and problems encountered during the four, eight-week tutorial periods of Phase II are grouped according to the basic organ systems. Because of the clinical experiences of Phase IB, students enter Phase II with a greater sense of what they need to know. They define their learning issues in greater detail and present and discuss cases within their tutorial groups with greater emphasis on patient management.

The final unit of Phase II, Unit 7, is designed by each student to meet his or her individual learning needs. After a general theme is established for the Unit by the tutorial group, each student, in consultation with the tutor, pursues self-identified areas of learning. This is designed to facilitate the transition from the tutorial group experience to the behavior that will be expected of students in the hospital during Phase III. Precision, clarity, and effective communication are highly valued. At the end of Phase II, students take Part I of the National Boards. Passage of this exam is a requirement for promotion to year three at the medical school.

Phase III. Much of the last two years of training takes place in a tertiary-care (hospital) setting. Students from both the PCC and regular curriculum progress through the traditional clinical rotations together. During the fourth year, PCC students are required to do a two-month primary care subinternship in a medically underserved area.

Figure 2.2. Sample schedule of student week during Phase IA of the Primary Care Curriculum.

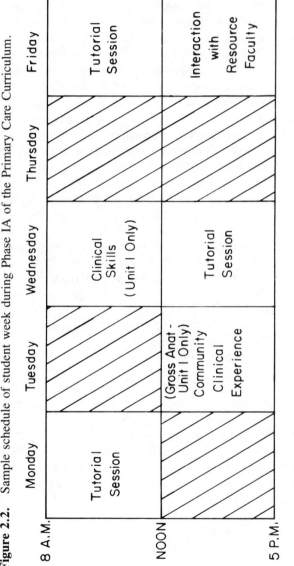

Major Types of Case Format Currently Used

During the on-campus Phases IA and II, students are exposed to a variety of problems which represent common clinical issues confronted by primary care physicians in New Mexico. The problems are presented in different formats including problems on decks of cards—P4 decks or PBLMs—simulated patients, paperpacks, and focused cases. Each of these formats is more fully described below.

1. *P4 Decks/PBLMs.* The P4 (Portable Patient Problem Pack) deck is an innovative case presentation format developed by Barrows and Tamblyn (1977). It is a deck of approximately 300 cards consisting of five color-coded sections each representing a different category of action available to a physician in working with a patient—history, physical examinations, laboratory investigations, consultants, and therapy. The specific category of question—examination, test, consultant, or treatment—is printed on the front of each card, and the answers appropriate to the patient problem appear on the reverse side. Each P4 deck includes all information available to the physician during one encounter, usually the initial office visit.

The PBLM (Problem-Based Learning Module) is a more sophisticated clinical problem presentation developed by Distlehorst and Barrows (1982).* Here the entire sequence of play is bound in two volumes, one a Master Action List, the other a Patient Encounter. The former is an alphabetical compendium of all possible historical questions, physical examination maneuvers, and diagnostic tests suitable for any patient problem. The latter is the particular patient problem broken down into responses to Master Action List inquiries. The PBLM is easier to handle than the P4 deck and provides less cuing of specialty areas pertinent to the patient problem.

2. *Simulated Patients.* The simulated patient (SP) is a healthy person who has been trained to portray the physical, emotional, and historical features of an actual patient. The SP is not meant to replace experience with real patients, but is a realistic learning resource for the development and refining of interviewing and examination skills.

The tutorial group agrees on a set of ground rules prior to encountering an SP, and this information is conveyed to the SP before the simulation begins. This includes:

1. The purpose for using the simulation (e.g., evaluation, interviewing techniques, physical examination).

---

*Information about PBLMs can be obtained from: Linda Distlehorst, Southern Illinois University, P.O. Box 3926, Springfield, Illinois 62705.

2. The size of the group and the format for the session (e.g., each student will interview, entire group will interview simultaneously).
3. Whether specific techniques are being emphasized which may highlight particular portions of the interview, the extent of the examination (i.e., pelvic, rectal, etc.), and an estimate of time required.

The SP format provides the tutorial group with an opportunity to reason its way through a problem using a "time-in" and "time-out" technique. This allows the student who is assuming the role of the doctor to stop the interaction with the SP ("time-out") and discuss questions and problems with the other members of the group. When the next steps of the interaction have been decided upon, the "doctor" declares "time-in." The SP resumes his or her role, and the encounter proceeds. The SP also provides verbal feedback. This is one of the few encounters with a patient in which the student will be told by the patient how he or she felt about the interview and examination—whether the student was comforting, seemed interested, asked appropriate questions, performed adequate physical examination, and so on. Simulated patients also complete a written feedback form when they are used in a formal student evaluation (see Chapter 8).

3. *Paperpacks.* Each paperpack is a written narrative of an entire patient problem. The problem is presented in segments of varying lengths. Each segment is immediately followed by questions designed to stimulate discussion of pertinent topics. This format emphasizes the ability to synthesize data, define underlying causes, and establish investigative and management plans without having to contend with the mechanics of the P4 deck or PBLMs or the emotional overtones of dealing with an SP.

4. *Focused Cases.* A focused case is constructed like a paperpack, but is generally very brief and emphasizes very specific problems or topics. They are occasionally used to assure that learning of specific ideas presented in one of the other formats has been thorough.

Historical Perspective

The PCC curriculum and choice of case format have evolved significantly during the past six years. Initially, aware of the almost magical benefits to learning expected from the small-group, tutorial method observed at McMaster University in Hamilton, Ontario, curriculum planners sought out the quintessential problem-based curricular technology of the day. They familiarized themselves with theoretical and experimental work on clinical reasoning by Elstein, Shulman, and Sprafka (1978), the key "how to" text on use of simulated patients by Barrows (1976), and the most avant garde patient problem format of the time, Barrows and Tamblyn's P4 deck (1977). Using these tools, the planners felt confident in adopting this new educational technology in toto.

Initially, all cases designed for the first two years of the program were in P4 deck format with simulated patients available for the history and physical portions of many cases. P4 decks were chosen because they allowed open-ended inquiry and freedom to pursue erroneous pathways, enabling students to learn by making mistakes. The P4 format had never been adopted as the basis of an entire curriculum, and New Mexico was to serve as a laboratory for their extensive use. During the final year of planning, a large number of P4 cases based upon the McMaster P4 prototype were prepared from patient charts. A cadre of simulated patients was also recruited and trained to match the symptoms and history appropriate to each P4 deck. The work was enormously time-consuming and often tedious. In addition, there was pressure to create a large number of cases to allow students to choose those cases that would best meet their own identified learning needs within each unit.

An initial problem in P4 case development was the conversion of the prototype P4 format developed originally for highly subspecialized problems (i.e., Neurologic), to a system in which primary care problems could be presented. Since primary care problems necessarily involve all organ systems and myriad diagnostic and therapeutic options, the number of cards in the P4 deck needed to be increased and headings for the cards as well as their specificity had to be significantly altered. The P4 development process began by surveying patient encounters in primary care practices. A list of 38 of the most common primary care problems was generated from these surveys, and a P4 deck was developed for each one. The decks were printed on computer cards so that the sequence in which a student chose the cards—the investigative and treatment approaches—might be coded for subsequent computer evaluation of the reasoning processes.

Whereas Phase IA focused on common medical problems, Phase II was organized around organ systems, largely for convenience of problem development and selection. The students' approaches to the P4 decks prepared for Phase II were expected to be far more sophisticated than in Phase IA. In Phase IB, the students would have acquired a clinical framework upon which to expand their understanding of clinical and basic science. Based on the experience of preparing P4 decks for Phase IA, the decks for Phase II were generated by having "case-writing retreats." Four or five clinical specialists would gather with clinic or hospital charts of patients with ailments identified as important by curriculum planners. Under the guidance of an expert curriculum planner, the clinicians would write case summaries, convert the cases to the P4 deck format, and generate a list of prompting questions that they felt would focus the students' attention on the scientific issues underlying the patient problems. In practice, however, many of these cases were not able to be placed into P4 deck format because of the pressure of time. These remained as paperpacks.

Feedback on the Initial Curriculum. Trends began to emerge over the first two years based on the accumulated feedback from students, tutors, and other faculty who voiced their concerns about the program's philosophy and execution.

Students returning from their rural experiences (Phase IB) complained about P4 decks and simulated patients. During Phase IA, students had been enthusiastic about the P4 deck and SP formats. After extensive exposure to real patients, however, these formats appeared too "artificial." The time spent wading through the cards and discussing the reasoning process seemed too tedious, and the amount of basic science material learned was too little for the time invested. They preferred to use real patients or brief problems generated either by themselves or by the tutors and curriculum planners.

Those who planned the initial PCC curriculum had assumed that students would learn all necessary basic science content adequately using P4 and simulated patient formats. The students, however, expressed great concern that their command of anatomy, microbiology, and pharmacology was inadequate. This was somewhat substantiated by their poor performance on these subjects on Part I of the National Boards. Students thus requested more focused introductions to these subjects.

This feedback created logistical problems for the curriculum planners. Relatively little time had been spent developing brief or focused cases, and those which were available did not cover all the student requests and were not of uniform quality. Newer cases of sufficient quality would have to be developed rapidly at a time when the number of students in the program had grown from 10 in the first class to 25 over two classes; and administrative demands on program planners seemed to be increasing exponentially.

Finally, both students and tutors complained that they had insufficient information to know which of the numerous P4 problems would best suit the needs of a particular student. Students also felt that they received too little feedback on the breadth and depth of their learning and on how well they were apportioning their time with each problem.

PCC Responses to the Feedback. A Curriculum Committee was created to modify the program. The members of the new curriculum committee consisted of two anatomists, a pediatrician, and a family physician. These individuals had each experienced most aspects of the program, had previously worked well together, and shared similar beliefs about how the curriculum should be improved. After reviewing the general philosophy of problem-based learning, they identified problems with the existing curriculum and instituted the following changes:

1. An *experiential* introductory week was instituted at the beginning of Unit 1 to expose the students to the concepts and methods of problem-based learning and small group interaction and to serve as a transition from teacher-centered to student-centered learning. Tutors were more directive during this week than they would become subsequently, to ensure that the students understood what was meant by the vocabulary and concepts of problem-based learning.

2. Case formats were altered in response to the feedback that they need not all be of a broad, "first encounter" type during Phase IA, but rather should be "focused" to lead the students to cover specific objectives. To address the deficit in pharmacologic knowledge, for example, new paperpack and focused cases were developed in which the diagnosis was given and the students had to select, and provide the rationale for, appropriate pharmacologic therapy.

3. The number of cases was reduced to those of higher quality with clear, stated objectives. These would be adequately reviewed by tutors before each unit.

4. The number of problems in P4 deck and SP formats was reduced, and new paperpack and focused cases were developed to meet identified needs.

5. Students now were offered access to all objectives with an option to either use them as a guide or neglect them. These objectives included chapter headings from basic science texts, more detailed objectives written by the UNM faculty, and the specific and well-organized set of curricular objectives provided by Southern Illinois University.

The original PCC planners were reluctant to share with students curriculum objectives from which case problems were derived. They feared that students would study the faculty-derived objectives rather than learning issues derived from their own curiosity. After several years' experience, however, the faculty did an about-face.

Considerable objection to this curricular redirection was voiced by some PCC planners wed to the timing and approach of the original P4 decks and simulations. These individuals suggested that the original formats were not being used properly, that the faculty was becoming too directive, and that the Curriculum Committee was reacting reflexively to student and faculty anxiety about National Board scores. However, support for change continued to grow from student feedback. Contrary to the expectations of the initial PCC planners, students did not seem to work as efficiently as had been hoped in IA, were not adequately prepared for IB, and had little interest in the old case format after they had been in the hurly-burly of real-life clinical encounters "in the field" during Phase IB.

The revised curriculum for Phases IA and II, which was implemented in 1982–1983, is shown in Table 2.1. A summary of the major theme of Units 1 through 7, and the number of cases and variety of formats used in each unit, is presented in Table 2.1.

The emphasis of Unit 1 is an anatomical survey of the entire body, that is, "where things are and what their major functions are." Gross, cellular, and biochemical levels are correlated in each case. There is a half-day gross anatomy session each week throughout Unit 1. Students dissect the structures most related to the problems being studied in their tutorial groups. Case problems, such as a gunshot wound through the thorax or cholelithiasis requiring cholecystectomy, guide the dissection in these sessions. The weekly clinical skills sessions, too, are correlated with the cases under consideration in the tutorial groups to further reinforce tutorial learning.

Unit 2 introduces major mechanisms of disease. Borrowing from Collins' innovative textbook on clinical reasoning, *Dynamic Differential Diagnosis* (Collins, 1981), problems are organized to fit the mnemonic VINDICATE, standing for the basic mechanisms of disease—Vascular, Inflammatory, Neoplastic, Degenerative, Intoxication, Congenital, Allergic (and Autoimmune), Traumatic, Endocrine (and Metabolic).

Unit 3, originally designed to provide groups of cases presenting with similar symptoms, was now designed to introduce major topics in microbiology and pharmacology. Affectionately referred to by students as "Bugs & Drugs," the creation of this new unit emphasizes the

Table 2.1. Summary of Main Emphasis, Number, and Format of Cases Used in Units 1–7 of PCC Curriculum

Unit	Emphasis	Number of Problems	Format
1	Introduction to the anatomy survey and function of the organ systems	18	Paperpack = 18
2	Introduction to the disease process ("VINDICATE")	6	Paperpacks = 2 P4 Decks = 4 SP = 3
3	Introduction to microbiology and pharmacology ("Bugs & Drugs")	11	Paperpacks = 11
4	Clinical problem solving in cardiology, pulmonology, and nephrology	10	Focus Cases = 10
5	Clinical problem solving in behavioral science, neurology, oncology, and occupational medicine	10	Focus Cases = 10
6	Clinical problem solving in gastroenterology, endocrinology, reproduction, and hematology	10	Focus Cases = 10
7	Advanced clinical problem solving	[a]	Student-generated cases

[a]Variable

degree of flexibility that PCC exercised in addressing a curricular concern within a somewhat skeptical faculty environment.

Phase II cases were reviewed and the number of "core cases" to be encountered by all students was reduced. The strengths of these cases were referenced to appropriate categories of learning objectives developed at Southern Illinois University (*Curriculum Objectives,* 1980) in an attempt to allow students to make more rational choices regarding the order in which they would encounter cases.

To facilitate the transition from tutorial learning to the more individual functioning expected of students on the wards in their third year, Phase II students were urged to choose their own problems for discussion rather than having the whole tutorial group study the same case during Unit 7.

Each student practices oral case presentation within the tutorial and leads a discussion of the case problem without other students having had prior knowledge of the topic, approximating the mode of presenting and learning on hospital rounds.

Other Formats. Several other types of learning experiences have been tried in addition to the basic problem formats presented above as a part of the continued experimentation that characterizes the PCC program. One of the most successful of these experiments is a semester-long series of problem-oriented pathology correlation sessions developed by Dr. Cooley Butler of the Department of Pathology at UNM. Phase II was chosen as the logical time to introduce intensive pathology input, in conjunction with the organ system–oriented tutorials of Units 4 through 7.

Two features of these sessions are designed to retain the atmosphere of student self-education. First, the lecture format is avoided as much as possible. Beginning with the initial session, the students are expected to examine and describe gross and microscopic specimens, make diagnoses, and infer etiopathogenesis from them. The knowledge gaps thus exposed are used as the basis for later self-study. The faculty assist the students by clarifying problems, prodding student memories, and guiding discussions in profitable directions, rather than providing most of the information as would be done in a traditional lecture format. The second feature is the use of case studies as the basis for discussion. These are made available to the students several days ahead of time. In preparation for class, students are expected to have developed diagnoses and studied the relevant pathogenic mechanisms. The issues raised by prompting questions are discussed in class. The faculty role again is primarily one of guidance and clarification.

Student acceptance of the course has been extremely positive. Most students consider that these sessions constitute a high point of their second year. They feel that numerous components of their prior exposure to medical science are integrated in a unique and rapid fashion. The faculty's avoidance of lecturing is judged to be very helpful in this regard.

Although the teaching format has been novel for most of the

involved faculty, all of them enjoyed it greatly. The usual observation was that the PCC students behaved, thought, and interacted with faculty more like residents than "typical second-year students."

Case Guidance.   Many students and faculty worry that students are "not getting the basics" or "not studying in sufficient depth." While this is often born of an insecurity among faculty in truly relinquishing responsibility for learning to the student, inadequate problem selection and development can magnify the problem. Problems can be designed that require students to plunge quickly into cellular or biochemical issues, or that require them to step back and assess psychosocial or community issues.

The initial problems in the curriculum must assist the student in becoming comfortable with the terms and tasks used in problem-based learning. These include problem identification, hypothesis generation, description of mechanisms to explain how the hypothesized causes of the problem can explain the presenting signs and symptoms, and generation of learning issues—those key areas of ignorance or uncertainty identified in the course of problem discussion. Initial patient problems should be both brief and focused to enable achievement of the above tasks within one or two sessions. The goal is to introduce the method, not exhaust every possible learning issue of a problem.

Case Examples.   The following sample problem was developed for students beginning problem-based learning. It is typical of cases encountered during the first week of the program.

CASE PRESENTATION

Zebulon Kincaid is a 66-year-old married man, retired from work as a "roughneck" in the oil fields. He is a 60-pack-per-year smoker living on a marginal income. After wining and dining a woman he picked up at a bar, he began sexual foreplay but could not sustain an erection. He then experienced a sudden onset of crushing, substernal chest pain.

The group lists and ranks the patient's problems and identifies hypothesized causes for each. For a typical outcome see top table, p. 31.

The group might devote most attention to the first problem, potentially a more life-threatening concern. Other relevant case history and physical examination information is available to the students as they try to learn more about the case problem. Supporting exhibits are developed for the case and include EKG tracings, laboratory values including "cardiac enzymes," and chest X-rays.

Problems	Hypothesized Causes
crushing chest pain	heart attack indigestion anxiety muscle strain

inability to maintain erection	psychological
	something wrong with the
	  normal mechanisms
	  (neural? vascular?)

smoking	peer pressure advertising addiction

Designers of the case problem can usually predict major learning issues students will pursue and prepare exhibits and resources accordingly. One group's issues were as follows:

Specific Issues That Focus Tutorial Learning on Patient's Main Problem	*Issues More Appropriate for Individual Learning*
What is a heart attack? What causes pain in a heart attack? Does it make a difference to treatment or prognosis which heart wall is injured? What structures under the sternum might be a source of pain? Which of the known risk factors for a heart attack apply to this patient? What are SGOT, LDH, and CPK and why are they elevated in a heart attack?	What is the gross and microscopic anatomy of the heart? What are the risk factors for heart disease? How does the nervous system sense pain? What causes impotence? What do extramarital relations have to do with heart attacks? What is the relationship between stress and heart function? What causes indigestion? How does normal cardiac electrical conduction work?

To ensure that students explore relevant histopathology as they work through the case problem, the case designers add an unexpected calamity to the patient's clinical course toward the end of the case problem:

The patient made an uneventful hospital recovery from his heart attack. On the way home from the hospital, Zebulon was involved in a fatal car accident. Autopsy included histologic sections of the heart.

Students are then provided with exhibits that include unlabeled color photomicrographs of gross and histologic pathology slides at several magnifications showing the histologic appearance of normal cardiac muscle, a recent myocardial infarct (MI), and an area of an older MI.

Another example of a Phase IA case that focuses on a problem currently causing great consternation in our society requires an exploration of issues that are as broad as lifestyles and social values, and that are as complex as the research frontiers of immunology. It is designed to occupy four to six tutorial sessions.

CASE PRESENTATION

You have received a call from Ted, a representative of "Common Bond," a campus-based, gay support group. He says there is growing concern within Albuquerque's gay male community about AIDS (Acquired Immune Deficiency Syndrome) which, they have heard, can cause severe infections, rare cancers, and death among male homosexuals. He asks whether you and your tutorial group would be willing to explain what is known about the condition to a group of gay men on the following Friday. This small audience is sophisticated, he says. It includes some pre-med students, science majors, and journalism students. He is sure that there will be some questions about the high risk of gay men contracting other infectious diseases such as hepatitis, giardiasis, and so on.

Because this is a recent medical problem, the etiology and ramifications of which are not yet entirely clear, the students must rely heavily on current research articles to supplement the information in basic texts in attacking this problem. Furthermore, because the problem will conclude with a discussion with a group of gay men, the students are motivated to read about issues concerning sexuality and gay lifestyles.

In preparation for this problem, a guide for tutors was prepared by faculty from the Departments of Microbiology, Community Medicine, and Psychiatry, outlining issues in their respective disciplines which they felt were pertinent to the case problem. This information helps prepare the tutors to better facilitate the group discussion and make them feel more comfortable with the important parameters of the case (Table 2.2).

To help the Curriculum Committee review and improve case materials, it is important that tutorial groups fill out case evaluation forms after working the problem. Sample feedback on the AIDS case is shown in Figure 2.3.

Multiple Case Problems That
Address a Common Theme

By the second year (Phase II), PCC students express increased interest in working with multiple clinical problems that illustrate a common mechanism of disease. If they have studied an issue in one case, they find an enormous satisfaction in applying that knowledge to a new situation. Thus, the curriculum planners have developed groups of brief, focused case problems centered on a particular clinical theme.

For example, the problem of jaundice is explored in Unit 6 as the students study the gastrointestinal system. Each student selects one of the brief case presentations and discusses the mechanism of jaundice production pertinent to that patient.

JAUNDICE CASE PACKET

To review your understanding of the basic mechanisms producing jaundice, choose one of the patients listed below and describe how he or she became jaundiced. Use the following guidelines for your presentation:

Write down your ideas about what might be the causes of or specific mechanisms responsible for jaundice in each patient. Use sketches where appropriate.

List the historical questions, physical maneuvers, and laboratory tests that you would use to establish the most probable mechanism of jaundice in each patient.

Predict the results you would expect for each question, maneuver, and test used.

Jason LaMark is a 32-year-old married computer programmer who is homosexual. He has experienced seven days of worsening fatigue, loss of appetite, and mild diarrhea.

A 56-year-old man has consumed large amounts of alcohol regularly for the past 30 days. He has mild edema and says he bruises easily.

A 14-year-old black adolescent was diagnosed as having sickle cell anemia. He experiences episodes of severe abdominal pain.

Table 2.2   Guide for Tutors

The primary focus of this case is to learn the clinical significance of the immune system by observing the devastating effects which can occur when portions of it have gone awry.

Immunology

Acquired Immune Deficiency Syndrome (AIDS) adversely affects how the body handles bacterial and viral infections and malignant cells. While the exact cause is speculative, attempts to understand the condition will inevitably lead the student into the broad subject of immunology. This should be the primary focus for the student's learning.

All students should learn enough basic immunology information to be able to answer or do the following:

1. Review the steps in the inflammatory process. Cite major differences between acute and chronic inflammation.
2. Describe differences in origin, products, and function of B and T lymphocytes.
3. Explain differences between Type I (reaginic), Type II (cytotoxic), Type III (immune complex), and Type IV (delayed hypersensitivity) reactions in terms of different cell types (T, B) and mediators of inflammation (antibodies, histamine, complement, etc.)
4. Explain T-helper versus T-suppressor cells in terms of function and how their dysfunction can cause disease.
5. What are the clinical presentations that would lead you to suspect that a patient has an immunodeficiency disease? How would the type(s) of infections(s) help you determine the kind of immune abnormality present?
6. Present a list of infectious agents/conditions which are likely to be associated with immune deficiencies.

Epidemiology

Since this condition bears features of an epidemic in certain populations (male homosexuals, Haitian refugees, drug abusers, etc.), the condition lends itself very well to a review of methods of population study. This knowledge can prime students for community health assessment in the next phase (IB).

Behavioral Science

This case provides an opportunity for students to interact directly with those living an alternative lifestyle. It permits the student to explore very personal issues of sexual practices, and to serve in the role of health educator. In their readings, students should learn something of the special nature of the role of physicians when caring for homosexuals. They can also review films and behavioral texts on human sexuality.

Figure 2.3. Sample evaluation form completed by tutorial group: AIDS case.

1. What were the best features of this problem unit (if any):

   THINKING ABOUT THE GAY LIFESTYLE & HOW IT MAY AFFECT BOTH SIDES OF THE PT-DOCTOR RELATIONSHIP WAS INVALUABLE. I ALSO THINK THAT INTERACTING WITH GAYS DIRECTLY DURING THIS PROBLEM WILL ALLOW ME TO BE MORE EFFECTIVE IN DEALING WITH THEM AS A PRACTICING PHYSICIAN. THESE SOCIAL & MEDICAL ISSUES COULD EASILY OVERLOOKED IF WE HAD NOT BEEN EXPOSED TO THIS CASE.

2. What were the worst features of this problem unit (if any):

   NOT BEING AS COMFORTABLE AS I HAD ANTICIPATED DURING THE INITIAL PHASE OF OUR MEETING WITH THE GAYS AND ALSO NOT HAVING ENOUGH TIME TO EXPLAIN AND ASK QUESTIONS ONCE WE ALL BEGIN TO OPEN UP.

3. What suggestions do you have to improve this problem unit: POSSIBLY HAVE MORE THAN JUST 2 GAYS PER TUTORIAL & ALLOWING MORE TIME TO SPEND WITH THEM (SAY- 2 HRS?) HISTO-SLIDES OR GOOD PHOTOS OF KAPOSIS SARCOMA & CHEST X-RAYS OF PNEUMOCYSTITIS PATIENTS COULD BE HELPFUL.

4. Please rate the following three areas concerning this problem:

	GOOD 5	4	AVERAGE 3	2	POOR 1
Presentation & Format	GCE	PA			
Content & Issues	PG,A, C,E				
Resources Available	PGA CE				

5. Please list resources used for this problem (i.e., texts, journals, AVs').

BASIC & CLINICAL IMMUNOLOGY — *4 ED. STITES, LANGE PUBL.*

HARRISON'S PRINCIPLES OF INTERNAL MEDICINE

PRACTITIONER - NOV. 80 - 1151-1156

J.A.M.A. - AUG. 82 - 756-759

SEXUAL PROBLEMS IN MED. PRACT. - 81-AMA PUB.

VIDEOTAPES: NCME # 277 IMMUNOLOGY, # 352 NCME # 401- RWM 100 p. 95 RWJ-709-HBB

SCOPE MONOGRAPH - IMMUNOLOGY

IMMUNOLOGY - MICROBIOLOGY REVIEW

NEW ENGLAND JOURNAL OF MEDICINE

SCIENCE - 21 JAN 83 - P. 271-272

BARRETT: ESSENTIALS OF IMMUNOLOGY

CDC - MMWR - VOL 31 #34 - 9-82

NM COMMUNICABLE DISEASE SUMMARY 9-82

NEJM - Vol. 307 #12 - 729-31

6. Please indicate faculty resources used during this problem (both basic science and clinical) the length of time involved and # of students.

FACULTY NAME	LENGTH OF TIME	NUMBER OF STUDENTS
DR. SEI TOKUDA	1.5 hrs.	5
DR. BILL LAFFERTY	1 HOUR	19
LOVELACE GRAND ROUNDS	1 HOUR	19
NON- FACULTY HUMAN RESOURCES =	45 MIN	5
PETER GEROW- PUBLIC HEALTH ADVISOR		
2 GAY VISITORS	1 HOUR	5

A 2-day-old infant was delivered at home two weeks prematurely. Her weight is 2012 g. She is brought to you by her worried father saying, "My kid sure looks yellow."

A 62-year-old woman with a history of "gallstone pains" complains of episodic right upper quadrant pains and some diarrhea.

Following the discussion of each case by a student, the group can turn to the actual data from each case as a way of providing feedback and of stimulating further discussion. Such grouping of related focused cases permits each student to present his or her own case in the tutorial. This also facilitates cross-discussion, since all students will have researched related topics.

This style of student learning and interaction prepares students for the upcoming hospital clerkships. There, each student presents his or her own patient to the rest of the ward team.

Role of Basic Scientists in
Case and Resource Development

Development of cases and supporting resources is a time-consuming, but central, task for the PCC program. The input of basic scientists is essential to both the academic and political success of the program. The original PCC planners, however, were clinicians who did not have daily contact with the basic science departments of the medical school. Dr. Stewart Mennin, an anatomist, was recruited to help involve basic scientists and basic science departments in the PCC program. He revived a dormant Curriculum Advisory Board composed of basic scientists and clinicians which had been formed during the initial planning stages of the program and changed it to a committee of Discipline Representatives who could act as liaisons between PCC and the various basic science departments.

One fear, voiced mainly by basic scientists, was that because the problem-based curriculum was open-ended, it would leave students with wide gaps in their knowledge. How could PCC ensure that students probed to sufficient depth in each problem? In order both to improve the program and to help the basic science faculty feel less alienated, PCC asked them for very specific help. Each department was asked to develop a core curriculum, and a questionnaire grid was designed for departmental input for each patient problem case. A sample form completed by an anatomy professor is shown in Table 2.3.

Yet a number of faculty complained that they received no feedback from PCC about the value to the program of their efforts. The initial response by the PCC program to this type of criticism was to require the students to keep a list of every resource used and every faculty member consulted. It was hoped that this could be used for purposes of review by external critics. Tutors were also asked to dictate summaries of each group session. This not only led to an administrative nightmare, tying up the office staff, but it failed to provide any meaningful measurement of learning.

Current efforts to improve the use of faculty input include the designation of specific individuals to be primary resources for each case. The tutors are instructed to urge the students to contact them whenever appropriate. The designated resource faculty are also asked to participate in the planning of new cases along with the Curriculum Committee. In this way the faculty members involved receive tangible feedback for their efforts.

What We Have Learned

1. It is important to vary instructional strategies and case formats. "The quality of teaching can be compromised by excessive dependence on some instructional strategies to the exclusion of others" (Jason & Westberg, 1982).
2. The core of student-centered learning is the freedom to pursue self-defined learning issues within a case. Therefore it is better to develop fewer, high-quality cases which can best achieve course objectives, rather than providing an excess of cases from which to choose—a rather minor "freedom."
3. The best teacher is experience. It is an important first step to experiment with problem-based learning formats in entire courses, in tracks within courses, or in course segments. Starting small provides experience with the method, a testing ground to improve one's approach, and serves as a model from which educators can draw ideas for their own courses.
4. We found it an enormous time saving to obtain sample case problems and varied case formats from other institutions when initiating our program of problem-based learning. It is easier to modify an existing case for your own use than to construct one from scratch. Case development is usually laborious, and it diverts attention from the most important task—instructing faculty and students in how properly to use case problems for student-centered, self-directed learning.
5. It is important to accompany case problems with sufficient resources (e.g., X-rays, photographs, slides, drug samples), both to bring case problems to life and to familiarize students with the full range of diagnostic aids and therapeutic options.
6. It is beneficial to faculty in a problem-based program to provide basic science educators with practical clinical experiences and to expose clinicians to basic science developments.
7. Tutors must be informed about the major objectives of each case used by their group and feel comfortable in working with

Table 2.3. Sample Questionnaire to Collect Departmental Comments Regarding a PCC Case

Name_____ Date_____
Time involved 40 Minutes

Fact No.			Department	Anatomy	Clinical Diagnosis	Shortness of breath
Key Term or Fact from Case	*Free Association from Key Term or Fact*	*In General, What Does This Discipline Have to Do With Your Discipline?*	*Can You Be More Specific?*	*What Is the Biological Context in Which This Fits?*	*Prompting Questions: Specific Q's for Student Self-evaluation or for Tutorial Use*	
1	Shortness of breath	Bronchoconstriction	Nature of airway smooth muscle in the structure of bronchial tree	What is the structure of the conducting system of lung?	Respiration; gaseous exchange	(1) Does airway smooth muscle show different structural features than do vascular or gut smooth muscle? (2) Does airway smooth muscle respond to comparable pharmacologic agents as do vascular or gut smooth muscle?
2	Pleuritic chest pain	Innervation of lungs & surrounding tissues	Referred pain	What are the pain pathways to lung, pleura, & related thoracic structures?		
3	Sputum	Origin of sputum	Mechanism of production of sputum contents	What factors influence ciliary movement of sputum out of lungs?		

			(3) What factors influence sputum production (i.e., smoking, environmental pollution, allergies)? Are there variable cell types in the sputum? What are the origins of these cell types?
4	Chest X-ray	Bronchopulmonary segments of the lung	Be able to identify the segments of the lung in an X-ray
5	Convulsion	Control of motor systems leading to convulsions	Influence of body temperature or regulation of control of the motor systems
6	Pneumatocoele	Relation of lung structure in response to this condition	What other factors of a structural nature might be associated with this finding?

the exhibits (radiographs, pathology slides, laboratory data) provided.

8. The teaching environment plays a major role in a student's learning experience. The physical layout should provide a comfortable learning environment, that is, pleasant tutorial rooms with ready access to resource materials (tools, view boxes, large blackboards, and bulletin boards).

Experience at Other Schools

The new tutorial-based medical school curriculum at Mercer University is similar to that of the University of New Mexico in that it is based exclusively upon patient problems. The initial curriculum design was heavily influenced by the prior curriculum development experiences of a number of the Mercer program's creators (such as Ralph Berggren from McMaster and Paul Werner from Michigan State's Upper Peninsula Program). The four-year curriculum is divided into five phases.

The original problem design and case selection for the first two phases of the program focused on the themes of "communication" (introducing the student to the problem-based learning method and to the communities of central and south Georgia) and "cycles, continuums, and homeostasis" (introducing the way in which the human organism responds to its environment).

As time of matriculation drew near, many new faculty (predominantly basic scientists) were being recruited. Since they were not part of the initial planning group committed to problem-based learning, it was essential to introduce them to the concept. These newer arrivals were exhibiting the now-familiar skepticism about teaching basic science in such a "loosely structured" curriculum (R. Berggren, personal communication, November 1983). Berggren and others thus invited the faculty in each basic science department to review the case problems to ensure that the same areas normally taught in a lecture-based course were present in the case problems. This helped calm the new, anxious faculty members. It also clarified, for the curriculum planners, the areas where there were gaps and where there was redundancy in the subject case matter covered in the problems. Another benefit was that many of the basic science faculty saw, for the first time, where their disciplines fit into the broad scheme of the program. The basic scientists' review of the case problems was carefully documented, and this information served as a vehicle for outside review and accreditation.

Nevertheless, this portion of the program underwent a drastic revision in response to student and faculty feedback. After the first class completed the first year, a major problem was noted by faculty and students alike. When the students began the third phase, in which problems were organized by organ system, the depth to which they could discuss the problems appeared limited. The students simply did not have sufficient molecular and cellular knowledge from which to ask more probing questions during study of the case problems. In response, the faculty rewrote cases in the first two phases, sharply reduced the number of case problems, and selected three introductory problems that focused on molecular biology (cholera, herpes genitalis, and diabetes mellitis). In another important redirection from the original curriculum, such problem selection was less concerned with common problems found in rural Georgia and more with learning issues best suited to students' learning of medical science at this stage.

Experimenting with a more focused and controlled problem format, each basic science department reviewed the cases and listed the knowledge areas they expected students to cover. For this information, tutors' guides were developed that provided the tutors with case issues and other reference material. For it was now believed by course planners that if the tutor was knowledgeable about the problem, he would be able to pose more provocative questions and better facilitate discussion.

The early results of this revised curriculum for the second Mercer class were universally assessed as positive. The conflict of ideas proved an important learning experience for the original curriculum planners. As problem-based learning "purists," they had believed that *any* case could serve the students' learning needs. Now they had to admit that the students' learning, in this system, might best be facilitated by a hierarchy of learning issues. Further, by having the courage to show flexibility, to compromise with more traditionally oriented educators, and to be open to learning themselves, the curriculum creators served as models for cooperative behavior and fostered an experimental atmosphere in which all could share the questions, contribute to the curriculum plan, and take pride in the results.

Michigan State University (MSU) College of Human Medicine offers students the option of two tracks—the traditional, lecture-based "Track I" and a problem-based, tutorial "Track II." Most of the behavioral and biological science content studied by Track II students is organized around a series of "focal problems" such as Anemia, Jaundice, Back Pain, Fever, and Dyspnea. As in the New Mexico program, gross anatomy was found to be a difficult subject to cover well in a problem-based curriculum. Thus, for logistical reasons involving availability of laboratory space and materials, Track II students take the standard anatomy course with Track I students during the first two semesters.

The MSU focal problems are perhaps the most structured curricular offerings of the problem-based medical schools. Each clinical problem consists of the following:

1. A basic concept list developed by faculty from different disciplines that the students are expected to learn while working on the problem. An example from the Jaundice Case series is as follows: Biochemistry concepts: (a) bilirubin, reference Harrison pp. 205–210, (b) bile acids, reference White pp. 60–61, 626–27, 1055–57.
2. A reference list of books, articles, and other pertinent material.
3. Two or three extensive clinical cases in which patient data are periodically interrupted by "STOP—THINK" questions to direct the student's interpretation of data or learning of key concepts. For example, a case synopsis in the Back Pain case series includes:

A 67-year-old woman presents with chronic, unremitting back pain, and you are the fourth physician she has consulted in the past half year for this problem. When you greet the patient, she ignores your handshake and complains about the long wait, her physical ailment, and the lack of help she feels she has received from the medical profession.

STOP—THINK
• What are some reasons a patient may manifest such anger?
• What might be an appropriate response to such a patient?

4. A content evaluation, with minimum performance standards, for each problem.

Jones et al. (1983) have responded to the questions arising from their highly structured approach to problem-based curriculum development:

Although the original planners of what became the Track II program preferred to keep the faculty-defined content to a minimum, thus allowing more individual student and group definition of learning objectives, this was not feasible given the nature of the college faculty, many of whom would accept the program only if the content studied and evaluated was essentially the same as in Track I curriculum. (p. 19)

While straying considerably from the high degree of student-centeredness originally envisioned, the MSU group believes that their high degree of faculty control may be more apparent than real. They find students' use of materials and attitudes toward different aspects of problem-based learning highly variable. For example, few students use the Basic Concept List as the primary focus of their learning. And while the cases are all written out as someone else's summary, thereby bypassing the data-collection process, they find that any simulations (including live patients and P4 decks) also have their reality limitations and are more costly and cumbersome than focal case problems. Further, as in New Mexico, they find that clinical experiences with real patients provide ample motivation and multiple opportunities to practice the techniques of medical problem solving.

Implications

No single problem format can satisfy all educational needs in a problem-based curriculum. It appears that students need variety in case-problem presentations for optimum learning and intellectual challenge. There can be brief problems, long problems, problem decks, simulated patients, and real patients. Selection of problem formats for development, however, must take into account the cost of preparation— large in simulated patients and problem decks, small in brief case problems.

While problem-based learning seems highly unstructured at first glance, it can be highly variable in its degree of structure. In fact, there appears to be an international movement toward more structure in the curriculum, with clearer problem objectives and better case focus to achieve specific learning objectives while maintaining the basic concept of a student-centered approach.

If the development of case problems and objectives is truly to represent an integration of different scientific disciplines, interdisciplinary faculty groups should develop the problem-based curriculum. This will facilitate the development of depth and breadth in the cases and attract a larger number of faculty to the methods and goals of problem-based learning.

References

Barrows, H. S. (1976). *Simulated patients* (2nd ed.). Springfield, Ill.: Charles C. Thomas.

Barrows, H. S., & Tamblyn, R. M. (1980). *Problem-based learning: An approach to medical education.* New York: Springer Publishing Company.

Barrows, H. S., & Tamblyn, R. M. (1977). The Portable Patient Problem Pack: A problem-based learning unit. *Journal of Medical Education, 52*, 1002–1004.

Collins, R. D. (1981). *Dynamic differential diagnosis.* Philadelphia: J. B. Lippincott Company.

Curriculum objectives (1980). Springfield, Ill.: Southern Illinois University.

Distlehorst, L. H., & Barrows, H. S. (1982). A new tool for problem-based, self-directed learning. *Journal of Medical Education, 57*, 486–488.

Elstein, A. S., Schulman, L. S., & Sprafka, S. A. (1978). *Medical problem solving: An analysis of clinical reasoning.* Cambridge, Mass.: Harvard University Press.

Jason, H., & Westberg, J. (1982). *Teachers and teaching in U.S. medical schools.* Norwalk, Conn.: Appleton-Century-Crofts.

Jones, J. W., Bieber, L. L., Echt, R., Scheifley, V., & Ways, P. O. (1983). *A problem-based curriculum—10 years of experience.* Presented at the International Conference on Problem-Based Learning, Maastricht, The Netherlands.

Miller, G. E. (1980). *Educating medical teachers.* Cambridge, Mass.: Harvard University Press.

Naisbitt, J. (1982). *Megatrends.* New York: Warner Books, Inc.

Pallie, W., & Miller, D. (1982, November). Communicating morphological cancers in healing sciences. *Journal of Biocommunications, 9*, 26–32.

Rogers, D. E. (1982, Spring). Some musings on medical education. *Pharos, 45* (2), 11–14.

Stuart, J., & Rutherford, R. (1978, Sept. 2). Medical student concentration during lectures. *Lancet, 2* Part 1, 514–516.

CHAPTER 3

Tutorial Groups in Problem-Based Learning

SUSAN M. LUCERO, REBECCA JACKSON,
AND WILLIAM R. GALEY

"Is he going to live?" Teddy's teenaged mother wore a pained facial expression as she gazed expectantly at Tim, a first-year medical student. She was chewing gum rapidly. "We're doing the best we can for him," answered Tim. "The doctors are working on him right now in the emergency room." He reached over and put his hand lightly on the sleeve of her torn jacket. "Can you tell me exactly what happened when you found Teddy on the floor?"

There was a long pause as Teddy's mother fixed Tim with her gaze, head still, mouth chewing continuously. "I don't know. It was like he just stopped breathing. Like he was all blue around his lips and his little fingers. He's not going to die, is he?"

There was another long pause. It continued. Tim was stuck. He exhaled, sat back in his chair, turned toward the other tutorial group members sitting around the table, and said, "Time out! Wow! How can I honestly answer her?" The woman simulating Teddy's mother took the gum out of her mouth and lit up a cigarette. Charlotte, another student in the group, went to the blackboard and said, "Let's see, from the clinic chart they gave us, let's write down Teddy's problems."

The group made the following list of problems and hypotheses:

1. *Stopped breathing—seizures? temper tantrum? respiratory obstruction?*
2. *Retarded development—congenital defect? maternal deprivation?*
3. *Discontinuity of care—poverty? lack of education? lack of transportation?*

They discussed which questions they could ask Teddy's "mother" to help distinguish among their hypotheses. This was especially helpful for Tim, who now felt emboldened by the multiple lines of inquiry generated from the tutorial discussion. He would ask whether she had had a fight with Teddy, whether her pregnancy and his birth were normal. He would ask how she felt about child care. He would ask about her upbringing.

Tim turned from the group back to the simulated patient. When he called "Time in!" she put out her cigarette, replaced the gum in her mouth, and fell back into character.

Goals

The tutorial group should provide an environment for the accomplishment of the following goals:

1. *Self-directed learning.* Students should use the group experience to stimulate their intellectual curiosity and encourage their pursuit of independent study.
2. *Clinical reasoning and problem-solving.* Students should be able to exercise the steps in clinical reasoning, from problem identification through hypothesis generation, hypothesis testing, generation of learning issues, and identification and use of appropriate learning resources.
3. *Communication skills.* Students should develop effective communication skills with respect to transmission of information and interpersonal interactions.
4. *Self and peer evaluation.* Students should become skillful in identification of personal strengths and weaknesses and those of peers, and should develop strategies for achievable improvement.
5. *Support.* Students should gain skills in appropriately using the group for emotional support, social interaction, and personal growth.

Introduction

Virtually all medical schools implementing problem-based learning are using the small-group tutorial as a vehicle. However, a great gulf can exist between how such a new program is designed and how well it achieves its objectives. Within an educational setting, the teacher is a critical variable. The preparation, orientation, and motivation of today's teachers must be understood by those introducing change in medical education. The degree of a teacher's support for change will depend on the congruence of that change with the teacher's views and vested interests. Only 21 percent of medical faculty have ever taken a formal course on the process of teaching, and only 39 percent have attended at least one workshop on education (Jason & Westberg, 1982). Further, few request assistance from educational consultants, and only a minority ever skim key journals on medical education.

Yet the development of effective tutorial groups in a problem-based learning curriculum may require a redirection of faculty attitudes. Where there was emphasis on the teaching of content, there must now be a willingness to gain skills in the facilitation of student learning— helping the student to integrate and use information, to solve problems, and to interact effectively in a group. The challenge, therefore, is to create a cooperative learning environment for students and faculty alike.

New Mexico Program

Getting Started

It was an eye-opener for PCC planners when, in 1977, they visited the problem-based tutorial programs at McMaster and Michigan State's East Lansing and the Upper Peninsula campuses. For weeks after the visits, New Mexico's emissaries mulled over their observations. They realized how important it was to help students identify the steps in clinical reasoning. A simplified summary of the steps in clinical reasoning is presented in Figure 3.1. One document from McMaster was universally embraced by PCC planners. It was a table comparing entering students' learning in traditional education with problem-based tutorial learning (Table 3.1). The table clearly capsulized the discrepancy between the environment of traditional medical education and the world of medical practice.

During the early years of PCC, the guiding principles of tutorial groups emanated from a mix of (1) close adherence to what had been observed at McMaster University, and (2) personal values of those

Figure 3.1.   Outline of the clinical reasoning process.

IDENTIFY PROBLEMS

GENERATE HYPOTHESES
OF
A. *CAUSES*
B. *MECHANISMS* by which causes create problems

RANK HYPOTHESES

TEST HYPOTHESES
A. Current Data and Knowledge
B. New Data and Knowledge

RE-RANK HYPOTHESES
(most likely hypothesis is tentative diagnosis)

TREAT
(to manage problems)

faculty administratively responsible for tutorials. However, in recent years, as a result of steady feedback from students and tutors in the program, the guidelines for tutorial function, tutor preparation, and student and tutor role expectations have both shifted and sharpened. Mounting external pressure on PCC to show results combined with the program's desire to proselytize elements of PCC among conventionally minded faculty led to a clarification of objectives and a resulting series of guidelines for tutorial group behavior.

What Happens in a Tutorial?

At UNM, each tutorial group is composed of five students and one basic or clinical science faculty tutor. Groups remain together for two months. They are then reconstituted with new tutors and a new, randomly chosen student mix. A typical group session lasts three hours, and there are three sessions a week for first-year students and two a week for second-year students. This schedule leaves considerable free time for students to

Table 3.1. McMaster's Comparison of Student's Learning in Traditional Education with Problem-Based, Tutorial Learning[a]

Traditional Learning	Problem-Based Learning
Schedule prepared by faculty; fairly tight.	Students largely responsible for own schedule, individually or in groups; unstructured schedule.
Competition with peers for "honors," for place in medical school, etc.	Encouragement to work cooperatively; sharing experiences, opinions, expertise, learning resources. Learning to be comfortable with saying "I don't know."
Main learning events: lectures, laboratory, recommended reading—with most students doing same thing.	Wide range of learning resources and events, many more than can be sampled by one person.
Manageable "chunks" of information small enough to be mastered for an examination.	Endless amounts of information, with emphasis not on mastery of information per se but on the management of information appropriate to each individual, and its application to problems.
Evaluation by end of course, examination, limited to defined "knowledge" objectives determined by professor.	Ongoing assessment of broad range of goals (including both personal and program objectives) with student as main evaluator of own progress.
Lecture room environment, with large groups of students	Few "class-wide" events; close associations with small group of classmates in tutorials.
Classroom environment, with large groups of students.	Several faculty educational roles, including the general tutor, the "resource person," and the student advisor roles.

[a]From "Information Brochure to Prospective Applicants," M.D. Program, McMaster University, Hamilton, Ontario, 1976–1978.

pursue independent study, work in the community, and meet with resource faculty.

What follows is a series of vignettes from one tutorial group working with a brief case problem during the early weeks of medical school. A typical case problem would last for two or three sessions. In this group the tutor, Bill, is a physiologist. He asked one of the students, Lisa, to read the case:

"Josie Martin is a 59-year-old woman with chronic, severe hypertension which is poorly controlled. She ran out of her hydralazine, hydrochlorothiazide, and digitalis one month ago, but didn't have enough money to refill the prescriptions. She now presents with marked dyspnea, diaphoresis, and leg edema."

Bill then asked another student, Paul, a quieter student, to go to the blackboard and be a recorder while the group made a list of the patient's problems. But before Paul reached the blackboard Caryn asked the group, "What do all these words mean—'dyspnea,' 'diaphoresis,' 'hydro'-whatever?"

Bill pointed to *Stedman's Medical Dictionary* on a nearby shelf and said, "Let's look it up." Greg took out Guyton's *Textbook on Medical Physiology* and summarized what he read on digitalis but said he couldn't find the words "hydralazine" or "hydrochlorothiazide." There was no pharmacology textbook in the room.

As a tutor, Bill felt that the group would miss the more central pathophysiologic issues in the case if they got bogged down in definitions so early, so he intervened. "Maybe we should just look up some of the drug names at home, and make them part of your learning issues for next session." The group agreed, and came up with the following problem list, which Paul recorded on the blackboard:

Student-Generated Problem List
1. Shortness of breath (dyspnea)
2. Diaphoresis
3. Leg edema
4. Chronic, uncontrolled hypertension
5. Poverty
6. Stopped medications

In the course of generating this list, the students argued whether associated social factors (such as poverty) or antecedent behaviors (such as stopped medications) should be designated as problems or simply be identified as contributing factors to the presenting symptoms. Bill encouraged this discussion, for the group was beginning to appreciate that management and intervention strategies could include many more options if social issues were included in the list of problems (e.g., "refer to social service" or "help patient apply for medical disability"). His role at this juncture was that of a mediator negotiating between students' competing ideas.

The students next spent a long time working on what they thought could be causing Mrs. Martin's problems. Here are two sample hypotheses from two problems on their list:

Problems	Hypotheses
1. Shortness of breath	Heart failure
	Pulmonary embolism
2. Diaphoresis	Fear or anxiety
	Pain
	Heart failure

Bill wasn't wild about this list, but recognized it as typical for students beginning problem-based learning. At first, students generate hypotheses, many of which tend to be specific diseases they have heard about (e.g., pulmonary embolism) rather than broader, underlying mechanisms (e.g., diminished oxygen delivery, airway obstruction, vascular obstruction). By keeping hypotheses broad and stressing underlying mechanisms over specific diseases, students learn the relevance of scientific understanding in clinical reasoning and are less likely to narrow hypotheses prematurely.

Now came a critical juncture in the session. Bill wanted to assess the level of understanding that the students had about the scientific issues in the case. He also wanted them to grapple with more complex scientific concepts in their study. He asked the students to take ten minutes and independently write out, to the best of their understanding, the mechanisms by which one of their hypotheses, fear, could cause two of Mrs. Martin's presenting problems—diaphoresis and dyspnea. On reviewing their work it was clear to Bill that the students' understanding varied greatly, ranging from Caryn's well-thought-out sequences to Peter's very elementary connections (Fig. 3.2).

The students reviewed one another's work, and asked one another a lot of "what if . . ." and "what do you mean by . . ." questions. Paul pursued Caryn's thought to the limit of her knowledge. He asked her where the respiratory center was located anatomically and whether the part of the brain which experienced fear could directly affect the part controlling respiration. She realized she didn't know. Paul discussed with Lisa whether adrenalin could directly stimulate sweat glands.

The students seemed wrapped up in the discussion, all but Peter. Bill tried to draw him into the discussion, but Peter either had little basic knowledge in this area or was preoccupied with an external problem, perhaps emotional. Bill would want to see how he functioned as the morning progressed.

As noon approached, Bill asked the group to summarize Mrs. Martin's problems. They discussed their understanding of those problems, summarized the central remaining questions, and made a list of

Figure 3.2.   A comparison of students' clinical reasoning.

CARYN'S REASONING:

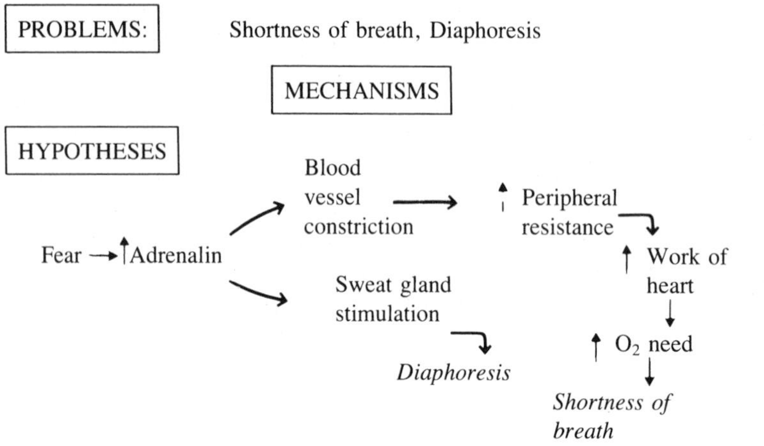

PROBLEMS: Shortness of breath, Diaphoresis

MECHANISMS

HYPOTHESES

Fear →↑Adrenalin

Blood vessel constriction ⟶ ↑ Peripheral resistance ↘

Sweat gland stimulation ↘ Diaphoresis

↑ Work of heart ↓

↑ O_2 need ↓

Shortness of breath

PETER'S REASONING:

Fear stimulates the heart to race and sweat to occur. The faster the heart beats, the more blood goes through the lungs, and this may cause rapid respiration.

learning issues that they would study before the next meeting in two days. The group listed the core issues all would study and the minor issues to be assigned to individuals.

Learning Issues—Mrs. Martin

All Will Study	*Individuals Will Study*
1. Control of respiration	1. Anatomic location of respiratory center—Caryn
2. Mechanisms causing edema	2. Relationship between adrenalin and sweat glands—Paul
3. Mechanisms causing hypertension	3. Mechanisms of action of hydralazine, hydrochloro-thiazide—Lisa

Bill thought their topics were too broad to be covered adequately in two days, but he decided to let them discover that on their own. Besides, they could always spend an extra session on the problem. He wanted to find a way to bring Peter into the group. He wanted to see Peter in a position of leadership, speaking out in the group. Maybe then Peter would feel more confident with the scientific material.

During the end-of-session evaluation, Caryn spontaneously said that she was disappointed that Peter hadn't contributed more because he "usually asks good, basic questions." She then asked the group if they thought she had talked too much. Paul said, "No, I like to hear you reason out loud—it makes me look at problems from a different perspective." Greg criticized the group's learning issues as being far too broad and said that next time they should ask more specific questions in their learning issues. Picking up on Caryn's point, Bill suggested that the next session begin with Peter presenting his understanding of the mechanisms controlling respiration and drawing them on the blackboard. Peter agreed and the group broke for lunch.

What Makes a Good Tutor?

Shaky Beginnings

After years of program development and critical analysis, it has become clear that in the initial phases of a problem-based learning program, no single element is as critical to program success as the quality and preparation of its tutors. However, the educational goals of a tutorial group and the ground rules for group interaction are unfamiliar to most medical school faculty. A skilled tutor must be a role model for students in such areas as quantity and quality of work, critical thinking, tutorial democracy, and enthusiasm and growth. The tutor should stimulate a high level of expectation and performance and facilitate the assumption of leadership skills by the group members. Such tutors are pivotal to a successful program.

Since tutorial group activity is necessarily intimate, highly interactional, and to a large extent student-initiated, its character is as varied and complex as the personalities and motivational levels of its members. "Rules" for tutorial behavior, therefore, are difficult to codify. They must allow flexibility and a wide berth for variation without jeopardizing the efficient functioning of the group or compromising the learning needs of all members of the group.

Initially, in PCC the concept of "student-centered learning" was held to be preeminent and inviolate. Consequently, a good facilitator was to be nondirective. Tutors were encouraged to ask nondirective questions, such as "Why do you say that?" and "Where are we going with this problem?" Directive participation was discouraged in order to permit "discovery learning" on the part of students who would thus gain "ownership" over acquired knowledge, study skills, and information-seeking abilities. Some tutors stuck so rigidly to this reflective, non-directive tutoring mode, that they withdrew from group participation to the point of being uninvolved.

In concert with this passive tutor model, students' group work on case problems was to be an open-ended affair, without limits on how much time students could spend with a given problem. The theory suggested that all medicine could be learned by studying any problem in sufficient depth. If students were enthusiastic about their learning, it was immaterial how long they dwelt on a particular issue.

Groups worked on different cases, at varied paces, and to unequal depths. Often the tutor would allow the students to drudge along with a case for many weeks, waiting for them to exhaust their interest or find their own way. The tutor may have withheld information which could have been shared with the group to focus their attention for a richer, more time-efficient learning experience. For example, one tutorial group studied a case of abdominal cramps for a full six weeks. They tried to learn every detail of the gastrointestinal system, totally losing sight of the relationship of this information to the patient problem in question. The tutor made only feeble attempts to go on to another problem. The fear of appearing too directive or lecturing to the students dissuaded many tutors from interfering, and they often felt they were in an educational and emotional straitjacket.

Suggestions for Revising the
Tutor's Role

By the third year of the program, discontent with the then current, loosely defined role of the tutor was apparent. The program staff reexamined the role of the tutor to determine which tutorial methods had been successful. Three steps were taken to collect data: (1) informal interviews were held with tutors and students, (2) the students filled out a questionnaire about the qualities of an ideal tutor, and (3) the information from students' evaluations of their tutors' evaluations was analyzed.

These data overwhelmingly confirmed that the students desired more active participation by the tutors. Students wanted tutors to offer more direction and critical feedback and to probe their understanding and clarify issues. Students who had experienced this type of tutor, as compared to the "laid-back" variety, felt that their sessions had been more motivating and interesting, and that they had learned more.

As a result of this reexamination, tutors and students in the first year were supplied with clearer, case-specific objectives. These provided more explicit time frames to work through the cases, to identify expert faculty resources, and to create questions that the group could use to help focus on particular problems that they could pursue in sufficient depth. New tutors were given a rigorous orientation to the principles of the program, as well as to the focus and objectives of the particular unit in which they would be tutoring. Ongoing support was given to the faculty members while they were tutoring, and guidance was offered to help them become more directive and interactive with the students who were entering this new type of learning environment. A greater demand was placed on tutors to learn their role. A document from the University of Illinois was invaluable (Table 3.2). It offered practical suggestions to tutors to help them facilitate clinical reasoning in the group. For the most part, our tutors are currently adapting to the new role, moving from that of lecturer/teacher to that of tutor/facilitator.

Background of the Tutor

Does it matter if the tutor is a basic scientist or a clinician? Is it better if he or she is an expert in the scientific field being discussed in tutorial? Students invariably value their tutors' ability to become involved in the group's learning and stimulate the group's enthusiasm. Such a faculty skill is either present or can be activated among basic scientists and clinicians alike. A tutor's special area of expertise can also be used as an asset for the group. For example, it is common for a group to praise a basic science tutor with, "I really appreciate Dr. W.'s tutoring style—he kept prodding us to explain clinical phenomena at the cellular level." It is equally common for clinical tutors to be praised with, "It was refreshing for Dr. K. to force us to make clinical connections with the physiologic and pharmacologic issues we were studying." One problem concerns the feeling of insecurity among many basic scientists when placed in a clinical environment. Some are almost paralyzed at first, fearing that they will appear foolish, unable to "lead" the group or ask the right questions. The reason this is not a common problem is that such faculty usually decline to tutor. They are happier and can make a better contribution to the program as a resource expert in the defined area of their interest.

It is often true that a tutor expert in the area being discussed by the group may be able to ask more probing questions and conjure up better resources for his tutorial. Yet expertise is freely available to tutors and groups in books, articles, and resource faculty. We have increasingly

Table 3.2. Practical Suggestions for Tutors to Facilitate Steps of the Reasoning Process and Problem Solving[a]

Summary

a. Tutor encourages analysis, synthesis, and evaluation of data.

b. Tutor encourages students to model his/her behavior in asking for reasons, justifications, etc.

c. Tutor intervenes appropriately to keep discussion on track, to give information, and to stimulate thinking.

Suggestions

1. *Tutor elicits students' reasoning process.* If a student asks for more information from the presenter (e.g., "Did patient vomit?"), tutor might ask "What are you hoping to find out? What are your reasons for asking that question? How would knowing the answer make a difference in your approach to the patient's problem?"

2. *Tutor encourages hypothesizing, asks for the reasons why specific hypotheses are suggested, and elicits evaluation of hypotheses.* Tutor might ask, "What do you think is going on with this patient?" "What *reasons* do you have for offering that specific hypothesis?" "What evidence would rule in or out these hypotheses?" One student suggested that tutor should ask, "What disease or other processes *could* have caused this?" rather than asking, "What caused this?" The student thought that the former approach would elicit many hypotheses to work through and evaluate.

3. *Tutor maintains continuity and focus of discussion by asking for periodic summary, by asking for evaluation about what has taken place, and by asking where the discussion is going.* Tutor might ask, "Will someone summarize what has taken place thus far?" "Who would want to summarize that presentation in 30 seconds?" "What would we look for now with this patient?"

4. *Tutor encourages students to make connections.* Tutor might ask, "What is the association between hypertension and headaches? How might interdisciplinary issues about patient lifestyle be related to this case?"

5. *Tutors emphasize open-ended questions to promote discussion rather than focusing on yes/no type questions or emphasizing quiz-type questions which are not integrated with discussion.*

6. *Tutors emphasize mechanisms and causes of patients' problems.* Tutor might ask, "What processes could have caused this problem? What are the mechanisms involved here?"

7. *Tutors periodically ask students to explain and define medical terminology used.* Tutor might ask, "What is cholesterol? What does that level of cholesterol usually mean?"

(continued)

(continued)

8. *Tutors do not simply answer all questions that are asked, but appropriately deflects them back to the group.* Tutor might ask, "Does anybody know the answer?" "How might we go about answering that question?" "What impact will the answer to your question have in regard to approaching the patient's problem?"

9. *Tutors encourage students to refine their presentations and make them more precise.* Tutor might ask, "How might you quickly summarize what you've been saying? What's a more precise way of saying that? How could you better organize that to get your point across more effectively?"

[a]From *Tutor Notebook,* University of Illinois School of Clinical Medicine at Urbana-Champaign, 1980–1981.

matched tutors with particular units on the basis of their expertise on the subject matter of the unit's cases. However, we do this as a recruiting device more for the comfort of particular tutors than the learning needs of the students.

An exciting development is the use of third- and fourth-year PCC students as tutors and co-tutors. Their contributions have been enthusiastically received by tutorial groups and the experience affords the student tutors an opportunity to gain teaching skills and review basic sciences.

Group Process

In small-group tutorials, students share their knowledge with peers and learn from a myriad of interpersonal experiences. Understanding the functions and processes of groups and group interactions is the core of making small-group tutorials effective. PCC's tutorial planners established three major functions necessary for an effective tutorial group. The following outline (here abbreviated) is distributed to the students at the beginning of the term:

1. *Use the group to develop effective communication skills.* It is important for everyone to communicate effectively. This entails communication not only of technical information, but also of feelings at the personal level. We come together with varying abilities to communicate, and it is only through active practice that we can improve these abilities. It is important that each member become an active participant in the group in order to contribute his or her unique knowledge and ideas to the learning process.

A. *Transmission of information.*   You will have the opportunity to present information to the group in a variety of
ways. Each of you will be expected periodically to
present and summarize information about the patient
from the case, just as you will have to do as a practicing
physician. You will also have the opportunity to present
concepts and newly acquired information to the group. It
should be emphasized that these are not envisioned as
"mini-lectures" or "show-and-tell times." Rather, they
should be delivered as succinct personal communications tailored to meet the needs of the group.

Another function of communication is to formulate
appropriate questions relevant to the case. In our experience, questioning is one of the most important means of
facilitating learning, not only for the individual asking
the question, but for the group as a whole. It can serve to
keep the group focused, and prevent it from getting
bogged down. It also can help other group members by
forcing them to present information and concepts more
precisely. The only question that can be considered
"stupid" is the one that is not asked.

B. *Interpersonal interactions.*   It is essential that the tutorial become more than a cold, pragmatic assessment of
medical cases and information. We all communicate
more effectively when we can open up with our true
feelings and share "who we are." Not all of us have
developed the skill to communicate feelings and personal
concerns to a group in a manner that provides for constructive resolution. Any group of people who work
together closely and consistently will have to address
problems in the areas of leadership styles, listening abilities, and giving constructive criticism and feedback.
Learning these skills can be as difficult as mastering
complex scientific disciplines.

2. *Use the group to assess the performance of the group, peers,
and self.*   We need to be able to assess ourselves, our peers,
and the group as a whole in four areas: (a) learning of basic and
clinical science information, (b) use of reasoning processes,
(c) identification of appropriate informational resources, and
(d) use of communication and evaluation skills.

These are some of the most important and difficult areas
that must be dealt with in the tutorial. It is next to impossible

to grow as professionals or individuals without honest and open assessment of our skills. Others are usually reluctant to give us open criticism unless we actively encourage it and honestly desire to receive it. And unless we really want to be evaluated by others, their comments can often be ignored or misunderstood. Criticism need not be construed as a personal attack. To lessen the likelihood of that occurring, criticisms should be given in a context of caring and honesty and should address only appropriate and specific items that can be changed or modified.

3. *Use the group for support: Emotional needs, social interaction, and personal growth.* The tutorial is a small group of people with common interests and concerns and similar goals. It provides a unique opportunity for individuals to provide and receive support in several areas common to a person's well-being. Opportunities often arise for individuals within the group or for the group as a whole to administer to emotional needs. It also provides opportunity for social interaction and the development of friendships. Finally, through its openness and caring, the group can enhance the personal growth of each individual.

Group Time versus Individual Time

In a tutorial program, students spend most of their school time on work outside the tutorial. Students study independently at home, work in the library, consult resources, and review individually and in groups. Since only six to ten hours a week are actually spent in the tutorial group, there is a great mismatch between the substantial amount of material the student has studied and learned outside and the small amount the student will have time to present and discuss in the tutorial. This can be a considerably disappointing introduction to problem-based tutorial learning. The students feel that their efforts are not sufficiently acknowledged, their work not evaluated. Some students express insecurity about the loss of the more traditional reward of being tested on a defined area of study.

Unaccustomed to so much unscheduled time, a few students wallow in such freedom rather than using it for effective study. For them, informally structured activities such as scheduled resource times, group study, or sitting in on conventional track lectures provides a useful framework during the early transition from teacher-centered to student-centered learning.

Two particular tutorial methods have been found to be very helpful in improving the efficiency of students' tutorial experience and individual study time and in acknowledging students' individual study subject preferences.

First, at the end of each tutorial session, the study objectives for the interim before the next meeting are clearly defined. This improves the focus and efficiency of each student's study. Then the group decides which case-derived learning issues will be studied by all members of the group, and which by individuals alone. This is an extremely important group activity. It ensures that the tutorial group will discuss topics that the students have covered and enables each tutorial member to compare and assess the quality of resources obtained and the degree to which each group member grasped the topics.

Second, when the tutorial group convenes, it is useful for the tutor and students to review in brief the specific topics which each student covered. This is not only a matter of courtesy, but immediately involves each student in the discussion and gives some recognition for the work that was done.

Use of Resources

Early in a tutorial program, students are required to develop skills in selecting and evaluating resources. A tutorial meeting room is usually cluttered with texts, journals, medical dictionaries, and models, which the students have brought to illustrate a concept or support a particular point of view. Initially, students are guided in their trial and selection of different resources by the medical center library, and by a small, peripheral library where PCC students can browse through sample texts before deciding on which ones to purchase.

An early task in tutorial groups is to guide each student toward a personally suitable pattern of utilizing resources. In a tutorial group the very different learning styles and, thus, resource needs of group members quickly become apparent. Some students discover that they approach problems best by first reviewing basic texts to provide a framework upon which later detail can be added. Others can more easily infer general principles by starting with more complex materials such as research articles. There are students whose orientation is best fulfilled by audiovisual material, or face-to-face discussion with a faculty member or fellow student.

Considerable group discussion centers upon which resources students found most helpful. Consequently, substantial development of resource selection skills occurs among the students. PCC's methods of evaluation (Chapter 8) place great value on these skills.

While students soon become adept in the use of inanimate resources, they find it very difficult to use faculty resources. PCC planners found this surprising. They had envisioned a community of scholars—faculty and students—in which there would be an easy flow of information.

Although the students quickly felt at ease with their tutors, most shied away from faculty who were not in PCC. The students felt that their questions were too elementary to bother the faculty. PCC had initially cautioned their students to seek faculty resources only after they had researched their questions thoroughly. This was a precaution to avoid bothering faculty members who might already feel overburdened and add to the problem. Surprisingly, outside faculty criticized the infrequency with which PCC students consulted them—some faculty misinterpreted this humility as arrogance.

The difficulty of communicating was not one-sided. There was a pervasive discomfort among basic science faculty when they *were* called upon as consultants by PCC students. A frequently voiced complaint by these faculty was that "I find it hard to give an answer because I'm not certain what they have been exposed to and what they know." These faculty felt comforted and better oriented if they knew that a student asking a question had taken a particular course. This would provide a foundation upon which to structure an answer. Although this was a problem for some basic science faculty, it did not trouble the clinicians, who were not being called upon to change roles.

PCC planners responded to these communication problems by the active introduction of first-year students to the faculty at large. "Brown bag" lunches with basic science and clinical departments were set up to introduce PCC students to the expertise of each faculty member and to allow students and faculty to become acquainted in a comfortable environment. PCC invited faculty consultants into the tutorials, recruited more basic science faculty to work with students as consultants in clinical skills (Chapter 5), and emphatically encouraged students to seek faculty consultations independently.

Tutor Training

Formalized tutor training is a component of almost every problem-based medical school. During the early years of the program, lectures to potential tutors about their roles as good facilitators occupied much of the PCC tutor workshop time. Insufficient time was spent in giving potential tutors hands-on practical experience with the method.

Currently, a tutor training workshop is conducted over three days. The following list illustrates the topics covered via brief discussion, information packets, and practice sessions:

1. Philosophy of problem-based learning.
2. Clinical reasoning process.
3. Role of the tutor.
4. Evaluation and feedback.
5. Conflict management.
6. Phases groups go through.
7. Techniques of questioning, probing, facilitating.
8. Use of resources.

One tutor instructor works with three to five tutor trainees and an actual PCC student tutorial group. In place of lectures, theoretical concepts are allowed to emerge naturally (facilitated by the tutor instructors) during the practice sessions.

First, tutor trainees form their own groups and work with the tutorial case problem as students themselves. This provides insight into the method and a better appreciation on the part of the tutor of the actual task of the student. Tutor trainees then work with their student tutorial group for two sessions using the same case problem with which the trainees have just worked.

Each trainee spends about 15 to 20 minutes tutoring the group while the other trainees observe the interaction behind a one-way window. Trainees and students then offer each other feedback on their performance as major themes of the workshop are identified and discussed.

How Students Feel about Tutorials

PCC students generally express a strong allegiance to the tutorial method. For many, the skill of functioning productively in tutorials developed over time.

> *"I enjoy the small groups. We've become a supportive unit of people in a noncompetitive atmosphere. I really appreciate learning the differing points of view."*

> *"I was concerned at first about my self-motivation. I was mostly anxious about areas I didn't like or that were hard for me. But after*

the first two months, getting used to the process, I've learned to budget my time and pursue learning related to our case."

"I have learned the most about my interpersonal skills. The interactions in small groups can be a struggle in that it takes a lot of energy. But a lot can be revealed about one's strengths and weaknesses."

"What's really important to me is the feeling *I get, that* high *from figuring something out. When I would sit in lectures in college there would never be any thrill of discovery for me. The scientists were the ones who had experienced all that excitement 20 years before, and now I was just memorizing the results of their discoveries. But in PCC the* student *makes the discoveries and says, 'Wow! Look what I figured out!' Even if everyone else in the group already knew it, it's still a new discovery for the student. So there are light bulbs flashing all the time."*

Some students were uncomfortable with the tutorial method.

"Sometimes all the emphasis on group process gets in the way of our learning. I've had tutors who think the tutorial is supposed to be a group therapy session. I don't buy that."

"I came into PCC because I thought it would offer me a lot of independent learning. Instead the tutorial group really dictates a lot of what I have to study."

"Tutorial groups never gave me an adequate background of information on a subject. They never gave me a method for studying. They never sat me down and said, 'This is the subject and these are the readings to get you oriented!' So I felt lost a lot of the time because I need someone to give me that framework. I would struggle through ten pages of a chapter and barely understand it while_____would have read the entire book with full comprehension. I'd feel awful. My self-confidence took a nosedive."

PCC's tutorial group methods have a special meaning for many of its minority students.

"Minorities have always been told that they're inferior, they don't do as well on national boards, MCATs, and other tests. You can't help but feel that maybe you don't stack up if all our scores look so bad. But I think that PCC gives me a little kick in the butt to get my own priorities in gear and my own medical education in focus

*rather than the same old thing of being led down the lane by
somebody else.*"

"*The most beneficial aspect of PCC has been my increased
familiarity with the language and terminology of medicine. As an
undergraduate I could follow lectures but couldn't use the terms
and vocabulary. In PCC I have developed the confidence to express
myself verbally. I have to explain things to my classmates in tutorial
so that they can understand. This requires that I use the right
terminology.*"

"*Navajos think about things a lot before they do something. They
weigh things a lot. For example, when someone dies in a Navajo
family, there is no will. Everyone gets together to discuss how
things should be done. Another example is that there are chapter
house meetings for tribal government. At these meetings people sit
and weigh things. So sitting back and looking at problems makes
sense to me. Trying to determine what's involved and what to do is
just what we do in PCC. I see my father doing the same thing taking
care of the cows when they are ill. PCC fits better for me.*"

How Tutors Feel about Tutorials

Tutors usually have strong, positive feelings about the experience.
Participating in small-group learning allows them to know their students
well, and to see at close hand a student's feeling of exhilaration about his
or her learning.

"*In the tutorial, I got a much better appreciation for the way
students think. It made me appreciate the way physicians think. . . .
Basic scientists tend to be more factually oriented and less con-
ceptually oriented. What the students are doing in a tutorial is more
valuable to them. . . . I saw them working hard, freely putting
things together in ways that were meaningful to them. I think that's
the reason they enjoy it so much.*"—Biochemist

"*Tutoring is an intense experience, emotionally involving. I became deeply involved with the students. I think you have to, to be a
good tutor. It's a kind of interaction often missing from other
interactions with colleagues and friends. And I began to explore a
whole new avenue of interpersonal relationships in my own life. I
think I've changed tremendously.*"—Anatomist

"*[In the conventional track] every once in a while there will be
something that happens during a series of lectures that will make
you feel good, but for the most part you don't really look forward to
anything different. You know it's your turn to lecture, and, if you've
done it long enough, you basically know what to expect. There*

really aren't any great surprises, and you don't get to know the students very well. PCC offers a surprise element. You just don't know what's going to happen and it provides a certain sense of excitement and enthusiasm."—Physiologist

What We Have Learned

We have learned that the best teacher is experience. Faculty wishing to learn problem-based tutorial methods would do well to begin by practicing the technique on a modest scale—using small groups of students on their home turf. It is beneficial to observe how other schools conduct tutorials and to bring in consultants, especially if they can conduct a demonstration of tutorial learning. However, the giant step is taken and the most valuable lessons learned when interested faculty try their wings and run their own tutorials.

There is a variety of suitable tutorial settings in any conventional medical school environment. For example, small student groups could meet several times a week in parallel with any basic science lecture course. They could be guided by faculty who use case problems to encourage students to relate didactic material to real-life problems. Similarly, groups could form around case studies in physical diagnosis. An alternate approach to initiating tutorial learning is to experiment with a small, separate track within a particular course.

It is surprising how infectious the method is, how lessons learned from one experience modify and improve the next. To build a constituency it is critical to consciously bring in new faculty to try the method and offer feedback. It is almost impossible to predict which faculty will eventually embrace the method and contribute significantly to its spread throughout the institution.

The following points were particularly important to us:

1. *Students must have control of their learning.* The excitement of problem-based learning depends upon the students' sense of discovery and ownership over what they have learned.
2. *Start small.* One can easily begin tutorial groups within an existing course, as an elective experience, or in a new course. There is no better teacher of the method than experience and no better way to convince faculty of the value of its methods than personal exposure.
3. *Remain flexible.* No mix of students and tutors learns best in the same manner. The optimum working relationship between group members must therefore be negotiated. Each group

should expect there to be periodic adjustments in its rules and expectations. To retain a rigid set of expectations may hinder individual and group creativity.

4. *Tutor training should include tutor monitoring.* The skills of facilitating problem-based, student-centered learning are acquired slowly over time. It requires repeated practice with periodic critiquing by others skilled in the tutorial method.

Experience at Other Schools

The three-year M.D. program at McMaster focuses upon analysis of problems as the main method of acquiring and applying information. The fostering of independent study and the use of small tutorial groups are the primary learning vehicles in the first two years of medical school (Neufeld & Barrows, 1974).

Because problem-based learning is the primary mode of learning, all faculty must have at least some familiarity with this educational methodology. The role of tutoring is both accepted and widespread at McMaster.

Nevertheless, after more than a decade of experience, many faculty have sought changes in the program (Neufeld, 1983). Six issues have served as an impetus for change:

1. The expanding knowledge in human biology and health care.
2. Lack of clarity in program objectives.
3. A sense of neo-orthodoxy which some feared was building resistance to change.
4. A need by faculty for an infusion of energy and interest.
5. Difficulty in perceiving differences between McMaster graduates and those from other institutions, in the areas of integration of diverse skills in patient care, lifelong learning, and critical appraisal of clinical literature.
6. Insufficient exploration of newer technological learning resources.

McMaster faculty, students, and graduates explored these issues over a 12-month period. Three central recommendations, uncanny in their parallel to New Mexico's experience, were made:

1. Prepare a document stating the overall program goals and expected achievement by students at various points in the program. For example, this includes a description of key

concepts to be learned and skills to be acquired in a given problem. This document could be used to guide both student learning and faculty planning.

2. Revise curriculum units to introduce new concepts. A particular focus will be a new integration unit of cases to bridge the first two years with the third, clerkship year.

3. Assist students in their critical thinking skills. This approach was developed by the Department of Clinical Epidemiology and Biostatistics. Using clinical journal articles as a vehicle, students are challenged to make qualitative judgments about the new information presented, while gaining and applying statistical skills and refining their reasoning process.

Maastricht Medical School in Holland has experimented with various types of tutors, monitoring subsequent student performance (P. Bouihuijs, personal communication, November 1983). Those running this program have even tried upper-level medical students as tutors. They currently use both basic scientists and clinicians as tutors. They have compared tutors who are expert in the subject of the case problems to those who are not. While they have found student performance to be unrelated to the background of the tutor, students clearly prefer expert tutors. Bouihuijs suspects that since students spend only four hours each week with their tutors, they "want every moment to count."

The University of Newcastle Medical School in New South Wales, Australia, has been using the problem-based method of education for five years (Cox & Ewan, 1982). To help students work through a case problem, tutorial groups are stopped at appropriate points to generate hypotheses, apply students' knowledge, and determine their learning needs. Thus, the tutor is provided with a clear picture of the flow of reasoning. Each case is accompanied by a document that includes a list of successive steps in the problem, a reasoning procedure, a series of prompting questions, a listing of supplementary learning materials (e.g., anatomical renderings, biochemical charts, videotapes), and a number of test questions on a formative assessment.

This method of closely guiding tutorial groups in their reasoning processes indicates the degree to which problem-based learning can achieve specific learning objectives.

Important innovations in problem-based learning have been introduced into individual courses at Southern Illinois, Colorado, and Harvard. Southern Illinois University has introduced problem-based tutorial learning into their organ-system competency-based curriculum. For example, Richard Coulson, a physiologist and head of the ten-week cardiovascular respiratory block in Carbondale, wanted to change his course. He sensed a destructive competitiveness between students with an exaggerated focus on memorizing content as well as excessive faculty control of learning.

He decided to change his course to a problem-based tutorial format. He recruited fellow faculty in different departments to be small-group facilitators and to serve as expert resources. He then collected relevant case problems developed elsewhere and selected those most appropriate to his course. Students are organized into tutorial groups of six, which meet for about two hours, three times a week. They are expected to explain and understand case problems in terms of basic anatomic, physiologic, biochemical, and behavioral mechanisms. Students approach the problems cold, without prior lectures or a book of objectives.

Few faculty were enthusiastic at first, and many students were disgruntled with a block of study so discrepant with the objectives-based, faculty-directed format to which they had become accustomed. However, Coulson demonstrated that students in the new format mastered the same subject content as did students in the conventionally organized course the previous year (Coulson, 1983) and that tutorial-based students not only derived almost all of the pertinent case issues that consulting faculty identified from the cases, but explored many more as well. After three years of refining the course, there is mounting support from faculty and enthusiasm from students, who are now given an orientation to the method from the beginning of medical school.

At the University of Colorado School of Medicine, Ellen Tabak and Dr. Carlos Martini have led a team of educators in the development of an alternative track within the required Introduction to Clinical Medicine (ICM) course. The course meets one half-day per week and spans the first two years of medical school. Over the past four years Tabak and Martini have selected 14 students per year out of the class to pursue an alternative, problem-based tutorial track within the course which integrates basic and clinical sciences and emphasizes preventive medicine and early clinical experience in the community. The track has served as a training ground for faculty to learn the tutorial method and has generated other interest in the method within the medical school.

The physiology course under Dr. Clyde Tucker now includes a problem-based option for half the class during its cardiovascular portion and Dr. Jack Nolte, acting chairman of anatomy, has established an experimental, problem-based track within his neurobiology course.

In the spring of 1982, Dean Tosteson proposed the New Pathway track for the Harvard Medical School. One of the Harvard planners, Jeff Berman, a senior student taking a year off to help develop the New Pathway, worked with consultants from New Mexico's PCC program in establishing a "field trial" of problem-based tutorial methods to give Harvard faculty hands-on experience. He organized an elective course for first-year medical students which integrated clinical skills with pathophysiologic principles. All learning emanated from case discussions of four patients with the following diagnoses: nontropical sprue, rheumatic heart disease, chronic bronchitis, and nephrotic syndrome. There were two tutorial groups with six and seven students each which met two to three times a week. Two tutors guided each session, and other faculty who had written the cases served as expert resources to the group during the case wrap-up.

Student and faculty response was overwhelmingly positive. One student summarized the feelings of many,

> *"How refreshing to let our minds run free. There wasn't the pressure of learning to know the right answer. Instead we were encouraged to think and be creative—to use what little we did know in order to learn more."*

Berman's project has provided the critical first step, in a school planning to implement problem-based method, of translating theory into practice.

Implications

Students who come from conventional institutions and enter problem-based tutorial programs require considerable time and practice in learning the steps in clinical reasoning and in functioning productively in a tutorial group. Many problem-based tutorial programs have exhibited an initial tendency toward a loose tutorial structure. However, it was subsequently discovered that an ambience of ill-defined objectives and a reliance on self-directed learning undermined the fulfillment of program goals. Efficient student learning is facilitated by early institution of tutorial structure, teaching of steps in scientific reasoning, and guidance in tutorial interaction. This initial, structured orientation for students permits later, responsible assumption of tutorial learning skills.

The role of the tutor is critical for optimal tutorial group function. Since this role is often alien to faculty members accustomed to teacher-centered education, a carefully planned, hands-on, tutor training program must be developed.

References

Cox, K. R., & Ewan, C. E. (1982). Problem-based learning. *Medical Teacher*, *15*, 94–101.

Coulson, R. L. (1983). Problem-based student-centered learning of the cardiovascular system using the problem-based learning module (P.B.L.M.). *The Physiologist, 26*, 220–224.

Jason, H., & Westberg, J. (1982). *Teachers and teaching in U.S. medical schools*. Norwalk, Conn.: Appleton-Century-Crofts.

Neufeld, V. R. (1983). Adventures of an adolescent: Curriculum changes at McMaster University. In C. P. Friedman & E. F. Purcell (Eds.), *The new biology and medical education*. New York: Josiah Macy, Jr. Foundation.

Neufeld, V. R., & Barrows, H. S. (1974). The "McMaster Philosophy": An approach to medical education. *Journal of Medical Education, 49*, 1040–1050.

CHAPTER 4

The Library in a Problem-Based Curriculum

KATHLEEN SAUNDERS, DIANA E. NORTHUP, AND STEWART P. MENNIN

"I did my first year of medical school in a traditional curriculum, and my second in the Primary Care Curriculum. . . . In my first year, the only sources I used were class lectures, syllabi, and assigned readings from assigned texts. I never used the library, checked on an alternate source, went to the current literature. . . . I was not an exception. Very few students ever used the library. This year has been a totally new experience for me. My first task, I soon realized when I started in PCC, was to become comfortable with finding my own resources. . . . When I have a learning issue to explore, finding the resources myself helps me define the issues, the area of study, and what the disciplines are that need to be considered. Now when I have to study, I organize and define the areas of study myself."

Goals

The primary goal of educating students to utilize resources within a problem-based curriculum is to assist the students to develop skills for self-directed, lifelong learning. To this end, students must be able to do the following:

1. Interact effectively and efficiently with a complex and ever-increasing body of medical information.
2. Obtain library information in a timely fashion, selectively employing the variety of indexes, references, texts, audiovisual materials, and computerized resources that are available.
3. Organize and manage a personal medical data base which provides access to the information most relevant to their current learning needs and, ultimately, to their day-to-day practice of medicine.
4. Continue their self-directed learning activities during community-based portions of their curriculum.

Introduction

The library plays an important, central role in the problem-based education of medical students. The 1982 conference "The New Biology and Medical Education: Merging the Biological, Information, and Cognitive Sciences" identified "information overload" as one of the major problem areas to be addressed by medical educators (Friedman & Purcell, 1983). The conference recommended a shift from teaching students facts and information to helping students learn how to learn. One conference participant noted:

> The closest analog we have to the concept of "learning how to learn" is the skills we develop in using a library: we need to know how to get started, how to be efficient, what to keep and what to discard, how things are related, and where they are located. It is an active rather than passive role. (Strong, 1983, p. 182)

Little time is allotted for instruction in information management skills in most medical school curricula (Martin, House, & Chandler, 1975; Matheson & Cooper, 1982).

The information-searching process is one of the major steps in problem-based clinical reasoning (Neufeld & Barrows, 1974; Schmidt, 1983). Therefore, in many of the problem-based medical schools, the ability of students to identify and utilize appropriate learning resources is an established component of student assessment.

A source of major positive impact on the attainment of these research skills is the ability of the medical library to establish an active educational role in the problem-based medical curriculum.

The New Mexico Program

The 1977 Primary Care Curriculum grant proposed a medical school curriculum which emphasized self-directed learning and the development of skills for lifelong learning. Students enrolled in this curriculum would not take copious notes at lectures, read from faculty-prepared resource lists, learn the science of medicine discipline by discipline, or use the library primarily as a haven for quiet study. Instead, these students would identify learning issues and learning resources and use the library as a laboratory for interaction with a universe of medical information. They would develop efficient and effective information-seeking strategies for use over a lifetime.

A preliminary survey was undertaken to characterize students' study habits and use of resources in the problem-based and conventional curricula. A questionnaire was administered to ten students in each track in both the first- and second-year classes. Students were asked to record times and places of their study and list resources used, whether self-selected or recommended, over a four-day period during a representative portion of their curriculum. Seventy-five percent of first-year and 80 percent of second-year students completed the questionnaire.

Figure 4.1 shows that while students in both curricula study approximately the same amount of time in the evenings, the freer PCC daytime schedule is filled with more morning and afternoon study. The difference grows in the second year.

Table 4.1 reveals that first- and second-year PCC students spend a considerably greater amount of their study time in the Medical Center Library, compared to conventional-track students. While conventional-track students spent an increasing amount of time studying at home in the second year, PCC students spent more time consulting colleagues and resource faculty.

The questionnaire also revealed a marked disparity in the degree to which resources studied were either student-selected or recommended by faculty. In the problem-based track, 89 percent and 93 percent of textbook resources used were student-selected in the first and second year, respectively. In the conventional track, the figures were 26 percent and 27 percent.

In this initial study, PCC students relied less heavily on textbooks than did conventional-track students. In particular, PCC students used a

Figure 4.1. Distribution of study time between PCC and conventional-track students.

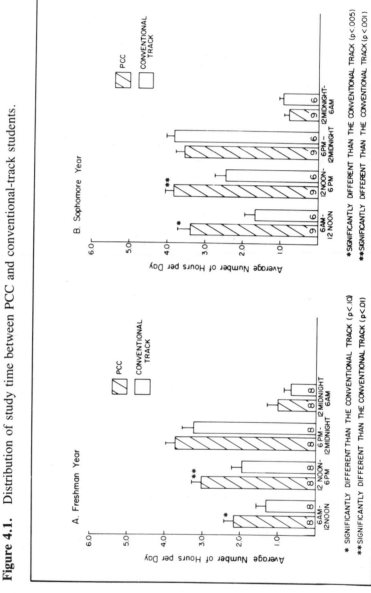

Note: Numbers at base of bars are the number of students completing the log of activities in each category.

74

Table 4.1. Where Students Spend Study Time

		Home	Library	Other
Year	PCC	47%	42%	11%
1	Conv.	49%	24%	27%
Year	PCC	45%	30%	25%
2	Conv.	71%	14%	14%

Note: Numbers may not equal 100% due to rounding.

larger percentage of journals (freshmen—24 percent of resources; sophomores—6 percent) than did conventional-track students (freshmen—9 percent of resources; sophomores—0 percent). PCC students also utilized a greater percentage of "other" resources (PCC freshmen 12 percent versus 6 percent for conventional track; and PCC sophomores 18 percent versus 12 percent for conventional track). The "other" category reflected an incredible potpourri of resources, including faculty, fellow students, patients, cadavers, a lecture by Dr. Elizabeth Kübler-Ross, a call to personnel at the Kidney Foundation, department seminars, conventional-track lectures and handouts, and a PCC student journal club. Conventional-track students' "other" category included notes, syllabi, faculty and peer consultation, laboratory results, and old exams. For the four-day study period, 17 PCC students listed 24 faculty consultations versus 14 conventional-track students' list of 5 faculty consultations. Additionally, these 17 PCC students listed 11 information searches (using an index, card catalog, bibliography, computer search, or reference librarian to locate information) versus no information searches listed for conventional-track students. Thus, during this study period PCC students utilized a greater variety of information resources.

Because PCC students self-select the great majority of their resources and use a greater variety of resources, early information search education assumes a greater importance within the problem-based curriculum than within the conventional curriculum. As a logical partner in implementing such a curriculum, the UNM Medical Center Library has become an active component of the experimental curriculum.

Education in Resource
Identification and Utilization

Information Search Education

In a 1980 address to the Annual Meeting of the American Association of Medical Colleges, the Dean at Harvard posed a succinct question regarding medical education: "Do we address directly the issue of how to find necessary information when it is needed?" (Tosteson, 1981). This issue *has* been addressed by the UNM Medical Center Library in collaboration with PCC since the very beginning of the new curriculum in 1979.

The task of assisting students to become efficient and effective information seekers has been difficult in the absence of established models. Over the years, UNM has tried numerous approaches. The first approach engaged PCC students in elective library tutorials modeled after the PCC tutorial process. A reference librarian guided the group through resources available for solving information problems based on a clinical case. This strategy was abandoned in favor of offering a series of separate instruction sessions which covered such topics as selecting textbooks, finding journal literature, using computerized literature search services, and organizing personal information files. Students were free to attend those sessions in which they were most interested. Goals and objectives of information search education are reproduced in Tables 4.2 and 4.3.

Additionally, librarians encouraged tutors to integrate the consideration of resources into the regular tutorial group process. Students who must regularly share the fruits of their information searches quickly

---

Table 4.2.   Goals of Information Search Education

1. Learn how to define and focus the information problem.
2. Understand the structure of the biomedical literature.
3. Understand how the biomedical literature is produced and know at what point the literature is likely to be useful to a specific information problem.
4. Learn how to evaluate the usefulness of a book or a journal article for a given problem.
5. Know how to locate material in the library.
6. Learn how to know which books, audiovisuals, and journal articles are appropriate to the problem.

Table 4.3.   Basic Skills Needed by PCC Students to
Find Information Effectively and Efficiently

Students need to know how to do the following:

1. Do a "quick and dirty" search for information.
2. Select and find standard textbooks.
3. Select and find review articles.
4. Find out if the library owns specific journals.
5. Identify appropriate audiovisual materials held by the library.
6. Use *Excerpta Medica, Index Medicus,* and *Science Citation Index.*
7. Use and interpret the *Medical Subject Headings* (MeSH).
8. Locate information on a topic not found in the above indexes.
9. Evaluate journal articles and books.
10. Identify appropriate resource faculty and community resources.
11. Differentiate when to do a computer search of the literature and when to do a manual search.
12. Organize materials (e.g., journal articles) into an efficient personal information file.

learn through the feedback of their peers and tutors whether the resources they have consulted and the strategies they have employed have been productive.

> *"The patients do not come with a list of readings around their necks."*

> *"Tutorial cases were most influential in my beginning to use journal articles as a regular source of information."*

> *"The library instruction helped show me what my information-gathering and decision-making patterns should be. As I went through the exercises, I found myself (1) thinking more logically and (2) reading the problems more carefully . . . to determine the most useful sources before I started looking for them."*

PCC has had, from the beginning, a librarian as a consultant in tutor training activities and as a participant in tutor meetings. In the course of formulating goals, strategies, and recommendations for information search education, UNM librarians identified two significant questions to be answered by the information seeker:

1. What are the elements of any information problem which may dictate the kinds of information resources to consult?
2. Which information problem elements favor one search strategy over another?

In an effort to assist the information seeker in answering these questions, Diana Northup, a UNM medical librarian, initiated a major project funded by the National Library of Medicine in 1981. The project had the following goals:

1. Identify categories of biomedical information problems of medical students, residents, and physicians.
2. Develop problem-based instructional tools, in the format of P4 decks (see Chapter 3), addressing these categories.
3. Use these instructional tools to teach the information-seeking process.

Northup's work, in collaboration with Umland and Bowermaster, resulted in the creation of the Information Searching Guides (ISGs)*, which are simulation tools used to teach medical students the process of finding information. ISGs present students with a clinical situation that generates the need for further information. For the information needs listed in the ISG, students choose information resources listed in an ISG Roster of Resources. The choices in the Roster simulate the possible resources available to a medical student. These include his or her personal library, the Department of Medicine Library, the Medical Center Library, the School of Medicine faculty, or the community at large.

After a student selects a resource with which to begin the information search, he or she turns to that resource in the body of the ISG. What the student finds is a synopsis of the information that would have been gleaned from the actual resource as it relates to the needs of the particular problem. Additionally, for each resource thus consulted, there is listed a time score (e.g., 45 minutes), which represents the time it would have taken to consult the actual resource; an efficacy score, which measures the value of the information obtained; and, if applicable, a monetary expenditure (e.g., the cost of a computer search of the literature). The student continues to consult the ISG resources until sufficient in-

*Additional information concerning ISGs may be obtained by contacting Diana E. Northup, Primary Care Curriculum, Basic Medical Sciences Building, University of New Mexico, Albuquerque, NM 87131.

formation has been obtained to satisfy the needs of the clinical situation. Students work through the ISGs individually, recording their time, efficacy, and monetary expenditure scores. After completing the exercise, a group of students, with a faculty facilitator, discusses the best pathways for the given type of information problem (e.g., finding information on very new phenomena).

Currently, five ISG information problems exist:

1. *Diagnosis and Treatment: Hirsutism,* which represents the search for standard, well-established diagnostic and treatment information.
2. *Subacute Bacterial Endocarditis,* which poses two information problems: finding pertinent, but somewhat general, basic science information, and finding very specific subject information.
3. *Drug Side-Effects,* presenting the search for very new information.
4. *Psychosocial: An Irresistible Urge to Steal,* which represents searching for psychosocial information.
5. *Patient Education: Multiple Sclerosis,* which emphasizes the finding of nontechnical medical information, especially from nontraditional information sources.

Preliminary evaluation of the ISGs at the University of Illinois–UC by Northup and Medin indicates that medical students using ISGs employ fewer steps in the information search and select better resources. Further testing is currently being conducted by Northup and Umland within the framework of PCC tutorials. First uses of the ISGs by PCC students met with a high degree of enthusiasm. After using the ISGs and following the group discussion of effective pathways, some of the students asked whether they could keep the ISGs longer in order to browse further. Additionally, students asked for copies of the Roster, to be used as a reminder, during Phase IB, of the variety of possible information resources. This testing will be used to determine how broadly the ISG can be integrated into the learning environment of PCC.

Personal Information Files

Research indicates that the personal library or reprint file is one of the most important sources of medical information for the practicing clinician (Northup et al., 1983; Stinson & Mueller, 1980). At the University of New Mexico, resources for assisting medical students, residents, and faculty in organizing personal filing systems are well developed. One professional medical librarian is responsible for all library consultations on organizing the personal information file (PIF). In addition, several Medical Center faculty and students have offered to discuss their filing systems with interested individuals. The basis for all PIF consultations is a printed guide entitled "The Organization of Personal Information Files in Medicine." This guide includes descriptions of alternative filing systems, their advantages and disadvantages, a source list of pamphlet materials, and an extensive annotated bibliography of articles describing methods of organizing personal files. It also poses practical questions and offers useful advice.

Five sample filing systems, complete with reprints, are available in the Medical Center Library for inspection and manipulation: a textbook-based system, a disease classification system, a cross-reference system, a MeSH-based system, and a homegrown system. In addition, the library maintains a collection of the reprints that are cited in the annotated bibliography of the PIF Guide. Finally, an Apple IIe computer and commercially produced data base management software are available in the library for individuals interested in evaluating the relative merits of a computerized personal filing system.

PIF consultations generally require no more than a single session of one to two hours. Students are asked to prepare in advance by reading the PIF Guide and having questions ready. Students in clinical rotations are also asked to record actual questions that occur during their work for which they would consult a PIF. This record is examined for patterns, which will be useful in determining the most effective framework for retrieval of information. This advance preparation is crucial to the productivity of the session. Students are also encouraged to bring to the consultation a representative sample of materials they wish to organize. There are no better examples than the students' own articles to illustrate the advantages and disadvantages of a filing system.

First-year PCC students are often particularly eager to develop a filing system during their initial weeks of study. It is difficult to convince highly motivated students to delay the establishment of a system until they have something substantial to file and until their interests and their frameworks for viewing medicine have gelled enough to provide the basis on which to decide upon a filing system. Students who are not yet familiar with a variety of textbooks and who have never seen a disease classification system are not quite ready to set up a useful personal information file. On the other hand, students about to embark on a rural clerkship in which they will rely heavily on journal literature should be prepared to organize a personal filing system.

Pervasive marketing of personal computers as effective information management tools has sparked a great deal of interest among medical students in the computerized PIF. While the current microcomputer technology possesses remarkable capabilities for information storage, retrieval, and manipulation, the computerized PIF is not necessarily a good initial choice for medical students. Few medical students have sufficiently extensive reprint files for the real power and advantages of computerized information retrieval to be readily apparent. Furthermore, the cost/benefit ratio of computerized versus small manual filing system can be questioned. The library's approach, then, is to assist students in establishing manual filing systems, while at the same time encouraging them to interact with the variety of computerized medical information resources available through the library.

PCC Student Library

Since the early days of PCC, a small library with various basic and clinical science texts has been housed in the PCC student lounge area. In addition, over the years, this library has been stocked with other resources, such as biochemical charts, portable anatomic models, and Kodachromes of histology slides.

The frequent student use of this library by PCC students confirms Northup's finding that physical proximity to resources is one of the most important determinants of their use (Northup et al., 1983).

Buying Books

In an integrated, student-centered, problem-based curriculum, students need to obtain a rather large collection of clinical and basic science reference books early in their medical education. As an illustration, the students' first biomedical problem during their first week of medical school concerns a dyspneic man. Learning issues derived from a discussion of this case problem could easily include topics in physiology, gross anatomy, histology, biochemistry, pathology, behavioral science, and medicine.

Since many students do a great deal of studying at home (see Table 4.1), a minimum purchase of seven extensive texts in the first week of school would be reasonable. However, this could be financially disastrous for students scraping through on loans. Therefore, PCC has made special arrangements with the medical bookstore to allow its students credit over a year's time.

Library Support for
Rural-Phase Students

By the time PCC students enter their rural clerkships, they have been involved for six months in a learning experience which demands heavy reliance on library resources. Yet rural medical practices cannot provide the extensive information resources to which these students are accustomed. Because PCC planners did not want rural practice to be viewed by students as professionally isolating, they emphasized the need for readily available library resources. Therefore, a major objective of library support for Phase IB is to enable students to continue their self-directed learning activities through easy access to the library by telephone or mail. Most requests are filled within 24 hours of receipt.

"I used more journal articles during Phase IB than I had used prior to that time. When I was in a town of 1,000, there I was reading the latest stuff. It would be there in my little post office box the day after I requested it."

To take full advantage of the services offered, an orientation to the procedures for requesting library services is provided for rural preceptors and students. This has been accomplished as part of a general orientation for all Phase IB participants just prior to the beginning of the clerkship.

The rural clerkship affords the student a perfect opportunity not only to use learning resources in the context of actual patient problems, but also to observe and evaluate the use of resources within the rural medical practice. And since most Phase IB students have just begun to organize PIFs, the clerkships allow the students to compare their own with their preceptors' filing systems.

The actual library support services provided to Phase IB participants are standard and straightforward:

1. Photocopying and mail delivery of journal articles.
2. Mail delivery of books and audiovisual materials.
3. Interlibrary loan of materials not owned by the library.
4. Computerized literature searches from which a librarian selects relevant citations to be photocopied and delivered with the printout of search results.
5. Reference services and brief subject searches to locate review articles, recent articles, or books on a well-defined topic.

One designated librarian serves as the liaison between the library and Phase IB participants. He or she interacts with library personnel, PCC students, and preceptors to solve service-delivery problems and also attends to special needs or complex requests. The following excerpts from one student's written request illustrate the demands on a liaison person:

> *"I am currently working on a PCC Phase IB Community Project involving a screening program to detect pesticide poisoning. We are dealing with cholinesterase inhibitors, specifically the organophosphate and carbamate insecticides. I need more information about the toxicology of these compounds and would appreciate the following material: [Citations for two textbook chapters] . . . and the relevant portions of [two textbooks and two articles, pages unknown].*
>
> *Now for the hard part: I would also like any recent references (if there are any) dealing with a comparison of the effectiveness of various cholinesterase activity testing methods, especially those comparing the Rappaport method to others; and also any current information on the effects of chronic, low-dose exposure to organophosphates and carbamates. Thank you for your help."*

What is unique about the Medical Center Library's approach to the delivery of services to Phase IB students is that library personnel have become attuned to the potential learning opportunities that exist in otherwise routine requests. When one student submitted a request for more than 50 articles from a computer printout, the library technician who received the request alerted the liaison librarian. He or she made use of this opportunity to initiate with the students a general discussion of the journal literature, types of journal articles and their relative usefulness for particular purposes, hints for selecting the best citations from a computer printout, and strategies for narrowing a huge literature base in any discipline.

During each four-month Phase IB period, the library fills approximately 400 requests for books, articles, and audiovisuals, executes about 40 computer searches, and provides an average of 40 reference and liaison services for 20 students and 20 preceptors. The PCC program absorbs the major costs of providing library support during Phase IB. The library charges its standard document delivery fee ($4/document) and computer search fee ($9/search) for provision of these services, but no longer recovers costs for reference and liaison services. In earlier years of PCC, the library received a total of $15,000 to support library personnel involved in the planning, implementation, and evaluation of library services for PCC, including Phase IB.

Preceptors obtain library support through the UNM Medical Center Library's Physician Outreach Program (POP), which extends library and information services to all New Mexico physicians for a yearly membership fee of $100. PCC purchases POP memberships for 20 Phase IB preceptors. Finally, students receive direct support from PCC for telephone calls to the UNM campus and for return mailing of library materials. Although this "communication support" represents a very small portion of the Phase IB budget, it is an essential ingredient in assuring that students are not inhibited in requesting and receiving information support services. The portion of the Phase IB budget devoted to current levels of library support amounts to approximately $4,500 per year.

Prior to 1983 PCC purchased POP memberships for its preceptors for the four months of the preceptorship. But in 1983 they began purchasing full, one-year memberships. Data currently available for the two months following the 1983 Phase IB indicate that the volume of preceptors' requests has remained high since the end of Phase IB. Thus, preceptors have used the library support not only during their Phase IB teaching activities but for their own continuing education activities.

A subject classification analysis of library materials requested by PCC students during Phase IB has indicated that roughly two-thirds of their requests are for basic science materials. This is a reasonably clear indication that students are able to continue learning basic science while engaged in an early clinical experience in an area remote from an academic library.

What We Have Learned

1. We can design problem-based experiences that facilitate students' development of effective and efficient information-searching habits.
2. It is beneficial to identify a liaison librarian to couple the unique learning needs of problem-based students and the resources of the library.
3. A legitimate function of the library is to provide assistance for students in designing and organizing their own filing system.
4. The library can instruct students in the clinical and scientific applications of information management and computer technology.

5. The library can serve as an easily accessible information resource for physicians remote from the medical center.

Experience at Other Schools

The introduction of such curricular innovations as problem-based learning and an extended rural experience has had a marked impact on the UNM Medical Library's programs and services. The Michigan State University (MSU) Libraries have had a very different experience. The first two years of MSU's problem-centered Medical track utilizes "focal problems" for which specific packets of assigned readings are made available through the MSU College of Human Medicine Clinical Center Library. Consequently, in contradistinction to the UNM program, there is little need for students to search for information and thus little need for formal interaction with librarians (L. Behm, personal communication, January 1984). MSU medical students spend their second two years in community-based clinical education away from the MSU campus. During this time, students utilize well-developed local hospital resources and rarely communicate with the science and clinical libraries on the MSU campus (J. Coppola, personal communication, January 1984). In contrast to the MSU experience, students enrolled in the Rural Physician Associate Program (RPAP) at the University of Minnesota (UM) are heavy users of the UM Bio-Medical Library, sending or calling in their needs from their rural sites (G. Foreman, personal communication, January 1984). RPAP's formal liaison with the Bio-Medical Library is strikingly similar to the goals of information services for PCC Phase IB and fulfills three objectives:

1. To provide information needed by students for study, research, decision making, planning, and patient care.
2. To acquaint students with an information-seeking method which will be applicable to rural medical practice.
3. To introduce students to the role of the librarian in the health-care delivery field. (Foreman, Wulff, & Verby, 1976, p. 201)

Special, conjunctive relationships between the libraries and problem-based medical programs also exist at McMaster in Ontario, and Mercer in Georgia.

As in New Mexico, students at McMaster receive no list of recommended textbooks, but are urged to use several before choosing one for purchase (Neufeld & Spaulding, 1973). McMaster has few formal lectures in its curriculum, so a large number of slide–tape presentations are offered. They are housed in the medical library, and many of them cover standard topics normally covered in lectures. Despite the enormous initial efforts to produce them, faculty have subsequently become disappointed at how little they are used. Virtually all of the information so painstakingly transferred to slides and tapes is readily available in texts.

A more successful innovation at McMaster was its laboratory modules in morphology (Pallie & Miller, 1982). Each of approximately 100 modules focuses on a theme in morphology, such as "endocranial compartments and meninges." The modules consist of monographs, slide–tape presentations, radiographs, videotapes, models, and prompting questions. By having concepts presented in graphic and three-dimensional modes, many students can more easily grasp the subject matter.

An important component of the curriculum at McMaster is the Critical Appraisal of the Literature Program. This program, initiated by the Department of Clinical Epidemiology and Biostatistics, guides students in assessing the value of information presented in the journal literature. An important co-requisite of learning to evaluate the medical literature is learning to find it. To facilitate the acquisition of information-searching skills, librarians co-tutor sessions in which the students are presented with a problem which they must investigate in the literature (D. Fitzgerald, personal communication, January 1984). During this investigation, students record the steps they take and use this record as the basis for a group discussion of information-searching strategies. A later tutorial focuses on the organization of a personal file and provides an opportunity for students to evaluate different systems before choosing one for themselves.

Librarians at the Mercer University School of Medicine make use of a variety of opportunities to instruct medical students in the search for information (J. Williams, personal communication, January 1984). Early in their first year, students are offered a potpourri of mini-workshops designed to teach basic library skills (computerized information retrieval, use of the card catolog, etc.). Librarians also serve as tutors, meeting with students once a month to focus on community medicine problems. These tutorials serve as an excellent opportunity for acquainting students with information resources and services.

The Mercer Medical Library received a grant in 1983 from the National Library of Medicine to develop a computerized network to support the information needs of medical students during their rural experiences. When complete, this computerized network will allow students from their rural sites to check the library's holdings and request desired materials, to request and receive computerized searches of the literature, and to obtain a file of experts who may be contacted for consultation.

Medical librarians at Mercer have participated actively in the development of the problem-based curriculum, participate in tutor-training workshops, and maintain an ongoing role in training medical students to be effective information searchers.

Implications

Implementation of a problem-based curriculum creates both greater demands and greater opportunities for innovative educational participation by the medical library. Early in their medical education, students need to obtain, store, and retrieve information efficiently. The library's range of assistance should be as varied as the learning needs of the students.

Since the educational program is geared toward skills in lifelong learning, the library must also seek innovative strategies to remain an active information resource for practicing physicians, regardless of their distance from the medical center.

References

Barrows, H. S., & Tamblyn, R. M. (1980). *Problem-based learning: An approach to medical education.* New York: Springer Publishing Company.

Foreman, G., Wulff, L. Y., & Verby, J. E. (1976). An information service for Rural Physician Associate Program students. *Minnesota Medicine, 59,* 200–202.

Friedman, C. P., & Purcell, E. F. (Eds.). (1983). *The new biology and medical education: Merging the biological, information and cognitive sciences.* New York: Josiah Macy, Jr. Foundation.

Martin, J. A., House, Jr. D. L., & Chandler, H. R. (1975). Teaching of formal courses by medical librarians. *Journal of Medical Education, 50,* 883–887.

Matheson, N. W., & Cooper, J. A. D. (1982). Academic information in the academic health sciences center: Roles for the library in information management. *Journal of Medical Education, 57,* Part 2.

Neufeld, V. R., & Barrows, H. S. (1974). The McMaster Philosophy: An approach to medical education. *Journal of Medical Education, 49,* 1040–1050.

Neufeld, V. R., & Spaulding, W. B. (1973). Use of learning resources at McMaster University. *British Medical Journal, 3,* 99–101.

Northup, D. E., Moore-West, M., Skipper, B., & Teaf, S. R. (1983). Characteristics of clinical information searching: Investigation using critical incident technique. *Journal of Medical Education, 58,* 873–881.

Pallie, W., & Miller, D. (1982). Communicating morphologic concepts in health sciences. *Journal of Biocommunications, 9,* 26–32.

Schmidt, H. G. (1983). Problem-based learning: Rationale and description. *Medical Education, 17,* 11–16.

Strong, H. (1983). Harnessing the information sciences to power the "new biology." In C. P. Friedman & E. F. Purcell (Eds.), *The new biology and medical education.* New York: Josiah Macy, Jr. Foundation.

Tosteson, D. C. (1981). Science, medicine and education. *Journal of Medical Education, 56,* 8–15.

CHAPTER 5

Clinical Skills: Enhancing Basic Science Learning

STEWART DUBAN AND ARTHUR KAUFMAN

The relationship between the basic and clinical [sciences] cannot be one-sided; it will not spontaneously set itself up in the last two years if it is deliberately suppressed in the first two. There is no cement like interest, no stimulus like the hint of a coming practical application. (Flexner, 1910)

Goals

The clinical skills course should do the following:

1. *Bridge the gap between basic and clinical sciences.* A clinical skills course should reinforce the relevance of basic sciences to the physician's clinical reasoning process and to the patient's history, physical examination, and laboratory evaluation.
2. *Place the student in active roles as "patient," "evaluator," and "provider."* Clinical skills instruction offers an opportunity for students to increase their awareness of a patient's needs by role-playing as patients for their peers, while observing and critiquing their peers' performances.

3. *Integrate the talents of basic and clinical scientists.*   Basic and clinical science faculty should plan and teach clinical skills together. Through such a collaborative effort, it is more likely that other aspects of the curriculum will begin to enjoy coherent goals and methods. Collaborative teaching also improves the environment for the faculty's own learning.

Introduction

Traditionally, clinical skills are taught only in the second half of the second year of medical school. They are taught solely by clinicians in preceptor format, with one to four students per instructor. There have been numerous modifications of the basic theme. For example, "Introduction to Clinical Medicine" courses have been spread over the entire first two years with the inclusion of much didactic material. Another approach has been the inclusion of clinicians in the didactic teaching of basic science courses, to illustrate the practical application of the basic science material. Despite innovations in clinical skills technology, basic and clinical sciences are still not taught in a related way.

Medical educators are beginning to recognize the limitations of presenting clinical science divorced from its basic science roots. For example, the revised Bates text, *A Guide to Physical Examination,* precedes each regional examination chapter with a brief, relevant "Anatomy and Physiology" discussion (Bates, 1983).

It is not surprising that traditional preclinical courses have met with only meager success in generating student interest and competence in the scientific basis of clinical practice (Jason, 1974). Historically, not only have the clinicians and basic scientists not pondered the design of such courses together, but they have often squabbled divisively over limited curricular time. Students' difficulty in retaining and applying basic science information while on clinical rotations is embarrassingly common. Clinicians grumble, "What were they learning during the first two years of medical school?" yet fail to sufficiently reinforce basic sciences on the wards. Basic scientists are often self-satisfied that they have discharged their duties and exposed students to the important material one or two years earlier yet fail to inquire how the information they have transmitted is retained or used on clinical services. The ball appears to be out of their court. Educators in a problem-based curriculum must, then, attempt to integrate clinical skills with their basic science underpinnings.

The New Mexico Experience

A clinical skills course was created for all first-year PCC students to reinforce the basic and clinical science subjects studied concurrently in tutorial groups. It is preceded by an "Introduction to Interviewing" course, which includes interviewing real patients. The clinical skills course focuses on the techniques of physical examination and the reasons underlying those physical maneuvers. History taking is reviewed in terms of the scientific rationale behind the review of systems questions.

To enhance the learning of clinicial skills, students practice physical examination both on classmates in the group and in community clinical settings. The course consists of one, four-hour session per week for 14 weeks beginning in the first month of medical school (Table 5.1).

Planning

Course sessions were initially planned by a basic and clinical science faculty team composed of two anatomists, a family practitioner, and a pediatrician. Over the past four years, this planning group has ex-

Table 5.1.   Schedule of Clinical Skills Sessions for First-Year PCC Students

Week	Subject
1	Overview of the general physical examination
2	Cardiovascular I
3	Cardiovascular II
4	Pulmonary
5	Abdominal
6	COMMUNITY CLINIC PRACTICAL
7	Male Genitalia/Female Breast
8	Female Genitalia
9	Neuromuscular I/Head and Neck
10	Neuromuscular II/Extremities
11	COMMUNITY CLINIC PRACTICAL
12	Laboratory—examination of urine and blood
13	Laboratory—microbiologic examination
14	COMMUNITY CLINIC PRACTICAL

panded. It now includes a second-year student, an internist, an emergency room physician, and a variety of basic and clinical science specialists who consult in their particular areas of expertise. The ingredient for success is simple: a mixed group of basic and clinical scientists who work comfortably together from the outset. Instructors from any discipline can contribute effectively to the planning of such a clinical skills course. Selected faculty can be invited to participate in individual sessions of the course. They must clearly understand the goals of the course and adjust their teaching format accordingly. A neuroanatomist might be invited to the neuromuscular sessions, a surgeon to the cardiovascular sessions, a microbiologist to the laboratory sessions, and so on.

The classroom courses, the tutorials, and the clinical skills course should be planned so that the order of the sessions complement one another. When the material is organized in this fashion, the student's clinical reasoning is more productive and satisfying.

Sometimes it is better to plan the order of the sessions in terms of basic educational concepts, rather than on the order of performance of the normal screening examination—head to foot. For example, as in Table 5.1, in the first week of school, we decided to present the cardiovascular system first because this system offers many generally orienting and unifying concepts which extend to each region of the body. Whatever order is chosen, the classroom courses or tutorials must be planned accordingly.

During planning sessions, attended by a core interdisciplinary planning group and a staff assistant, we generate a draft of ideas about what the planning group expects from the sessions. Notes from one of our planning meeting on the cardiovascular system read as follows:

1. *Medical history questions*

    A.   Identify the pertinent review-of-systems questions (e.g., "Do you get cramps in your calves with exercise? Have you had swelling of your legs? Do you become short of breath when you lie down?")

    B.   Generate basic science questions referrable to review-of-systems questions (e.g., "What biochemical mechanism underlies the phenomenon of calf pain when a patient with atherosclerosis of the femoral arteries takes a walk? What opposing forces determine whether fluid remains inside or outside capillaries? What mechanisms underlie the symptom of dyspnea when a patient with congestive heart failure reclines?")

2. *Physical maneuvers*
    A. Present an outline of motor skills (e.g., observe jugular venous pulses, palpate carotid and peripheral pulses, palpate precardium for location and quality of apical beat, auscultate cardinal areas of the heart).
    B. Generate basic science questions referrable to the physical examination maneuvers (e.g., "What physiologic forces comprise a pulse? What is the anatomic and physiologic basis of a valvular heart murmur? Why are "valvular" heart sounds loudest in areas away from their anatomic location?")

Following this draft of ideas, it becomes obvious that during the clinical skills session certain key concepts must be emphasized—the mechanisms by which venous blood returns to the heart, or the location, structure, and function of cardiac valves. An outline of underlying principles and clinical skills, including these new emphases, is then produced for distribution to students (Table 5.2). From this outline, a list of core questions is developed. Clinical-skills instructors are free to pose these questions to students as a guide to core concepts during the session.

We then identify supporting materials to which students or teaching staff might refer as resources to answer questions, illustrate concepts, or stimulate further interest. These include diagrams of metabolic or physiologic processes, photographs of normal and abnormal physical findings, normal and pathologic gross specimens, audiotapes (e.g., heart and breath sounds), animal organs for gross dissection, and histologic and pathologic slides with a microscope. Four sets of the material are packaged for each session—one set for each classroom. Use of the material is optional, and items are added and deleted frequently in accord with the students' reactions. A typical "resources" list for the cardiovascular sessions consists of the following:

1. Stethoscopes
2. Blood pressure cuffs
3. Ophthalmoscopes
4. Audiotape of heart sounds
5. Cow hearts with dissection equipment, gloves, and trays
6. PA and lateral chest X-rays of normal and abnormal hearts
7. Anatomic and physiologic heart illustrations
8. Three-dimensional models of heart
9. Full skeleton

Table 5.2.   Cardiovascular System

Principles and Skills (A Student Handout)

I.   *Principles*
   A.   Determinants of blood pressure.
   B.   Relationship of jugular vein pulsations to cardiac events.
   C.   Anatomic landmarks of heart chambers, valves.
   D.   Electrical conduction system, a sequence of events in the normal cardiac cycle.
   E.   Components of various heart sounds.
   F.   Determinants of cardiac output.
   G.   Physiology of a split second heart sound.
   H.   Starling's forces and edema.

II.   *Skills*
   A.   History
      1.   Principal symptoms of heart disease: dyspnea, syncope, chest pain or discomfort, palpitations, edema, excessive fatigue, cough, claudication, nocturia, orthopnea.
      2.   Important aspects of history: relationship of symptoms to activity; history of rheumatic fever, murmur, chorea, syphilis, thyroid disease; family history of congenital, valvular, or atherosclerotic heart disease; risk factors—hypertension, diabetes, smoking, cholesterol, diet, physical activity habits.
   B.   Physical examination

Components of Examination	*Motor Skills*
Skin—edema? cyanosis? arterial filling?	Observation & palpation
Blood pressure—reclining, sitting, brachial, popliteal	Palpation & auscultation
Pulses—arterial, venous, neck, extremities	Percussion
Heart—cardinal positions	Auscultation (bell & diaphragm)

Utilization of Resources

Anatomic models and mounted illustrations serve as important resources that elucidate concepts with which students are struggling. They complement the more time-consuming blackboard renderings by faculty who have variable artistic abilities. Traditionally, anatomic models are used almost exclusively in anatomy and pathology courses, but their use is equally functional in clinical skills sessions. Instruction in the performance of a pelvic examination, for example, is markedly enhanced by models of pelvic bones and illustrations of perineal and pelvic-floor muscle layers. The thoracic examination is aided by chest X-rays and by skeletons into which model lungs can be inserted.

Commercial resource materials can be very expensive. So beyond such basic items as skeletons, X-ray view boxes, and organ models we developed many of our own resources. The materials were inexpensively produced and are used by almost all of our faculty and students. The items are on display throughout a session, so that searching through books and stacks of charts seeking illustrative material is unnecessary. The photograph (Figure 5.1) illustrates the ready accessibility to students and faculty of myriad resource materials during a clinical skills session. Because each week brings a new topic and a new set of resources, a method was developed for easily exchanging resource displays from week to week. Course planners devised a picture gallery method for displaying photographs, charts, and diagrams. Thin strips of wood are nailed to the wall and lined with Velcro. Velcro patches are then affixed to the backs of sheets of cardboard onto which appropriate illustrations are pasted. Perishable resources, such as cow hearts, are obtained on the morning of the session from a local butcher.

The program is conducted in a contiguous, four-room cluster in the basic science building. This makes it easy for students in simultaneously run classes to share the one-of-a-kind resources—not only the expensive anatomic models, but also, at times, a single faculty consultant.

Development of Clinical Skills
Case Problems

Clinical skills planners have developed a series of patient problem vignettes that probe the students' understanding of major pathophysiologic concepts inherent in the session. Faculty have the option of offering them to students at appropriate times in the sessions. Examples are as follows:

1. If a patient has a systolic murmur, which valves might be involved (a) if the lesion was valvular stenosis? (b) if the lesion was valvular insufficiency?
2. During inspiration, what normally happens to pressure in the jugular veins and brachial arteries? Can you explain the mechanism for each?

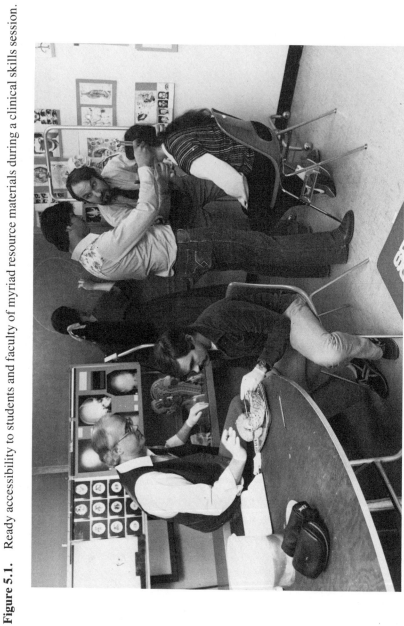

Figure 5.1. Ready accessibility to students and faculty of myriad resource materials during a clinical skills session.

Weekly Preparation Meetings

One to two days prior to the clinical skills session, there is a "tune-up" meeting of the faculty assigned to conduct that session. They review the planned skills and concepts to be taught and the support material to be utilized. The meeting provides an opportunity for the faculty to question each other about areas with which one or another might not be familiar. Basic scientists might practice the pertinent physical examination maneuvers and ask about their rationale. During one preparation session, for example, an anatomist was fascinated by the technique and rationale behind eliciting the hepatojugular reflux. Clinicians might review anatomic relationships or principles of pathophysiology. Clinicians frequently ask anatomists to review the embryology of the heart. They often ask physiologists to review hemodynamic principles. This review and exchange establishes a baseline of understanding among instructors to assist them in facilitating student learning.

Content of the Clinical Skills Sessions

The weekly session conforms roughly to the following time schedule:

Time	Schedule
8:15–8:30	Review objectives of the session
8:30–9:00	Practice previously learned skills
9:00–11:45	Learn new skills, correlation with basic science
11:45–12:00	Evaluate session (done by students)
12:00–12:30	Faculty discussion

Review Objectives of Session. A brief overview of the session is presented by one or two preceptors (usually clinicians). It often includes a clinical demonstration of the appropriate physical examination maneuvers. This is the only didactic portion of the session. However, even during the demonstration, the clinician may set the tone of the session by asking about, for instance, the location of the posterior superior limit of the inferior lobes of the lung, or the mechanism keeping alveoli inflated at small volumes.

Practice of Previously Learned Skills. A clinician/basic scientist faculty team can closely supervise clinical skills practice of two or three student pairs. With 20 students in each class in the problem-based track in New Mexico, the class divides into four groups—four to six students to a room. Students are free to choose partners for each session.

It was found that unless students practice newly acquired examination maneuvers from previous sessions, the maneuvers were soon forgotten or performed tentatively. Since repetition is a key to retention, student partners practice examining each other during the first portion of each skills session, using all the skills learned to date.

Learn New Skills.   Each student then performs the appropriate, newly demonstrated physical or laboratory examination with a partner, under close scrutiny by faculty, who offer substantial guidance. Students are encouraged by faculty to ask each other questions. When an impasse is reached, available resource materials and/or the faculty are consulted. Questions are also posed by the faculty throughout the session. An attempt is made to foster an atmosphere of openness and honesty as faculty and students share their ignorance as well as knowledge. "I don't know," is a common response in these sessions, on the part of faculty as well as students.

Enthusiasm for learning in depth should not be squelched by faculty rushing the students to "cover everything." Allowing students to pursue answers to their own questions enables them to learn at their own level at a comfortable rate. No one is held back, no one is pushed too quickly. What is important is that students make continuous links between the clinical and basic science fields and demonstrate an intellectual ability to move from a gross to a cellular understanding of observed events and posed questions.

PCC also places great value on faculty learning during the sessions. If faculty act as models for students, through the freedom with which they ask questions and expose their knowledge deficits, a more open learning environment is fostered. And when faculty are receiving new knowledge in the course of an educational endeavor, their own motivation to continue in the program is enhanced.

Evaluation of Session by Students.   The last formal part of the session includes an overall evaluation by the students. The results of these discussions provide immediate feedback to the faculty and course planners, enabling prompt improvements in the sessions from week to week. The importance of such a rapid reaction time by course planners in response to student input cannot be overestimated. It gives students a sense of true participation in course development and builds a sense of camaraderie and common purpose between faculty and students.

Faculty Discussion.   After the students have left, participating faculty meet to discuss the students' feedback. For example, the review might focus on the successful use of a short case which had illustrated a specific point and served as an excellent takeoff point for discussion. A specific resource might be criticized as being too complex for the particular concept the students were trying to learn. Notes from these meetings are kept by the course planners and incorporated into either upcoming sessions or plans for the same session the next year.

Other Sessions. Several sessions require additional description. The "Community Clinic Practicals" allow the students to apply their newly acquired clinical skills to the interviewing and examination of real patients. The first two sessions are held at two public schools and involve children entering the Special Olympics program. The third session takes place at a nursing home in which students perform full history and physical examinations on selected patients. In both settings, the impact of social, cultural, and economic forces upon the health and care of these particular patients provides an added dimension to the application of these clinical skills.

The "Female Genitalia" session enlists the aid of paid expert models, most of whom work in women's health care fields. They provide an opportunity for examination and offer feedback to the students. One first-year PCC student commented:

> *"The models gave excellent feedback, letting you know if you could probe further or if you caused pain or discomfort. It was one of the most informative sessions."*

While initially, students do not perform pelvic or rectal examinations on each other, many choose to do so after this formal session. During the "Male Genitalia/Female Breast" session, students select their own partners in mixed-sex student pairs and examine each other. Female students preferring not to serve as models can have paid models assigned to their group. Male faculty are always available as models, and male students seem less reluctant to be examined than females. One clinician who has taught in the clinical skills course each year summarized his personal experience with this portion of the course:

> *"The first year we tried this, I was really anxious and embarrassed. But I felt if we were asking students to reveal themselves to class-mates, it was only right that the faculty should demonstrate such openness themselves. So the other clinical faculty members demon-strated the male genital examination on me, while all ten students gathered around in nervous curiosity. The two anatomists got into the act as well—they had taught genital anatomy but never really did the examination. I was getting less self-conscious and in-creasingly interested in the teaching points. There I was, up at the blackboard trying to draw the varicocele that one of the students had discovered over my left testicle, when I noticed I had no pants*

on. . . . Soon, all of the male students were relaxed enough to be examined, and most of the women, emboldened by the risk-taking of their male peers, allowed their breasts to be examined. The same scenario has taken place each year. . . . You know, it's almost the turning point of the clinical skills course. Everyone's uptight before that session, but thereafter they are more relaxed, closer, and most trusting of one another. They've shared an important experience."

Following the clinical skills course, the students are provided with elective time—one-half day per week for four months—in order to further develop their clinical skills in the offices and clinics of community medical practitioners (Chapter 6).

Evaluation of Students' Clinical Skills

Informally, students are evaluated by peers and faculty within each tutorial session and while serving in the subsequent, community-based clinical electives. But also, every two months during Phases IA and II (five times), each student undergoes a formal clinical skills evaluation (Chapter 8).

Results and Rewards. The pairing of clinical and basic science faculty almost invariably results in important learning experiences for both. If a cardiovascular surgeon were teamed with a pharmacologist in a session, and the subject of cardiac rhythm disturbance came under discussion, the pharmacologist might provide much new information regarding, for example, calcium channel-blockers. Conversely, the cardiovascular surgeon might explain the metabolic and surgical causes of arrhythmias during open-heart surgery to both the students and the pharmacologist. Similar, complementary exchanges of information can occur between members of any such clinical/basic science team.

An anatomist who was centrally involved in planning and conducting clinical skills sessions summarized his feelings:

"I think it helps you as a tutor, helps you talk with medical students and other health professionals, because you now understand some of the basic medical skills. When you just stay within your discipline, do your assigned teaching of medical students, and then go off to your research, you get a very distorted view. . . . There is a need to know details of anatomy for particular purposes . . . but there is another anatomic way of thinking that is much more valuable to students. While most anatomy courses offer detailed regional dissection, [I now think] medical students' initial expo-

> *sure to anatomy should probably be on a systemic basis. . . . When you get involved with a whole clinical problem, you are always making correlations, and it puts your own discipline into perspective."*

This multidisciplinary approach to the teaching of clinical skills has also uncovered the lack of adequate textbooks for students struggling to integrate basic and clinical sciences. An effort to overcome this deficiency resulted in a successful grant application, to the National Fund for Medical Education, for PCC to develop an integrated, case-oriented text which stresses the use of basic science concepts in clinical reasoning. This type of clinical skills course is also one of the most efficient educational vehicles for demonstrating the value of problem-based learning in a conventional medical school environment. Every school already offers clinical skills instruction, and grounding such a course better in basic science mechanisms is appealing both to basic scientists and to clinicians.

The course has also influenced the conventional curriculum. A series of clinical skills sessions have been developed to complement the various regional anatomy portions of the first-year gross anatomy course. These provide a clinical context for traditional-track students. And multiple radiologic case studies with view boxes are now in place in the anatomy laboratory.

Problems. The major problems faced by clinical skills course planners relate to the course's large demands on faculty time. Participation is intellectually and emotionally rewarding to the participating faculty, but other department colleagues who do not participate often feel resentful that so much teaching time is diverting those faculty members from other traditional pursuits, such as grant writing and research. One participant lamented, "I feel frustrated because I feel myself being drawn [toward PCC] more and more, and becoming less connected with my own department."

The high ratio of faculty to students in this course presents another problem—that of student expectation. Clinical Skills is taught in the fall, the time of heaviest demands on most faculty. After an initial burst of enthusiasm by participating faculty, other demands gradually pull them away from the program. There are eight regularly attending faculty in the first session. By the later sessions, two to three months later, the number has been reduced to four or five. Students quickly become accustomed to the abundance of available faculty near the beginning of the course and are very disappointed by the relative scarcity in later sessions.

Future plans are thus directed at broadening faculty participation, yet at the same time decreasing the individual time commitment of each. The core, interdisciplinary faculty will be maintained. More faculty members than before will be asked to participate in the program, but each will be asked to participate in only two or three sessions.

What We Have Learned

1. *Students can profitably learn clinical skills early in their medical education.* A clinical skills course reinforces rather than diminishes student interest in basic sciences, if the course is presented in a manner complementary to concurrent basic science coursework.
2. *A clinical skills course may be the most successful vehicle for introducing problem-based learning into the curriculum.* Clinical skills instruction is the quickest, least disruptive method of introducing problem-based learning into a traditional curriculum. Since time is already set aside for such courses, the task is confined to emphasizing the scientific bases and the clinical reasoning which underlie clinical skills. Such a course will have wide faculty appeal for both basic and clinical scientists.
3. *Clinical skills learning is enhanced when basic scientists and clinicians serve together as faculty.* A productive dialogue between basic scientists and clinicians emanates from a common teaching/learning experience. Additional creative educational approaches then develop.
4. *Faculty members from many departments should be involved.* It is an error for only a few "believers" to be involved in the presentation of such a clinical skills course. Much valuable input from a large faculty group could then be lost. And further, the opportunity to institutionalize such cooperative teaching and learning among clinicians and basic scientists would be diminished.

Experience at Other Schools

Southern Illinois University (SIU) in Springfield provides its preclinical students with clinical skills instruction during their first and second years. The sessions complement the organ-system blocks of study, and it is intended that the students' skills build in complexity over the two years. In the first-year, cardiovascular block, the students learn a basic survey cardiovascular examination taught by a primary-care physician. In the second year, a cardiologist introduces the cardiac branching exam, discusses more complex neurodynamic issues, and brings in patients with cardiovascular disease.

For ease of instruction and supervision, SIU has constructed six examining rooms connected by entrances and one-way glass to a central observation room. The work of a number of students can thus be monitored simultaneously. Students practice clinical skills on fellow students, simulated patients, and real patients. This same economical arrangement of rooms lends itself to a unique series of clinical skills exercises. During the exercises each clinical skills room houses a different clinical problem. Students are given 10 to 15 minutes to interact with each problem and to demonstrate the requisite skills, including (1) interviewing, (2) technical maneuvers, and (3) clinical reasoning. One such vignette follows.

CASE PRESENTATION

The student is first given the following information before entering the station room:

The patient, Jim Gasparin, was brought to the Emergency Room by his wife after he had vomited blood earlier today. Mrs. Gasparin is in the room with him. Mr. Gasparin is 35 years old. Vital signs are

Temperature	97°F
Blood pressure	100/70
Pulse	112
Respiration	17

You are to gather information through interview and physical examination and arrive at some conclusions or plans for this patient. This is a busy day in the ER, so you have only ten minutes.

After you have taken the history and physical, pick up one of the sheets in the folder outside the room and answer the questions. You will have five minutes for this. Keep your sheet until the end of the exam.

The student then enters the examining room to find an ill-appearing man and his talkative, controlling wife (portrayed by actors). The man is made up to look jaundiced and even has small spider angiomata drawn on his skin. An emesis basin filled with "blood" sits beside his chair.

Students and faculty find the session lively and challenging. Moreover, the sessions closely approximate the actual time constraints placed upon clinical clerks and physicians caring for patients.

In an attempt to bridge the gap between the basic science curriculum and the realities of community practice, basic scientists at Morehouse Medical School in Atlanta, Georgia, are invited to the offices of community physicians to observe their practices (Kaufman et al., 1983). The basic scientists review medical records to determine exactly how basic science is applied in the actual practice of medicine. The chief complaints, problem lists, diagnostic techniques, and management plans are all evaluated. The basic scientists meet with the faculty clinicians, and together they analyze these diagnoses and management plans. The basic scientists then recommend curriculum modifications to reflect more effectively the relationship between basic science and ideal physician practice. For example, an anatomist observed a physician performing a pelvic examination of a patient in the lithotomy position. But students learn pelvic anatomy from the abdominal approach, on a cadaver. The anatomist realized the conceptual difficulties the students would have in translating from one position to the other. He therefore recommended that the pelvic approach be used on the cadaver.

In addition to basic scientists reviewing primary care procedures, primary care physicians review the curriculum of the basic science courses. They rate the relevance of the objectives of the curriculum to the everyday practice of medicine. A community physician noted that in the biochemistry course, three times as much time is devoted to the Krebs cycle as to acid/base balance and blood gases combined. Yet the latter are more useful to the primary-care physician. He therefore recommended that the emphases on these areas be modified accordingly.

Implications

Clinical skills can be efficiently learned from the beginning of medical school. The knowledge gained serves as preparation for early exposure to patient care. It can also correlate with concurrent coursework, generating a better appreciation for the clinical relevance of basic science subjects. Educational strategies can facilitate self-paced learning. Clinical skills education in the preclinical years can also serve as a forum for cooperative effort and shared learning between basic and clinical scientists. An innovative clinical skills course is the easiest avenue for introducing the principles of problem-based learning into a conventional medical school curriculum.

References

Bates, B. (1983). *A guide to physical examination* (3rd ed.). Philadelphia: J.B. Lippincott Co.

Flexner, A. (1910). *Medical education in the United States and Canada: A report to the Carnegie Foundation for the Advancement of Teaching, Bulletin No. 4.*

Jason, H. (1974). Evaluation of basic science learning: Implications of and for the GAP Report. *Journal of Medical Education, 49,* 1003–4.

Kaufman, A., Satcher, D., Jackson, R., Lewis, M., & Duban, S. (1983, Jan./Feb.). Undergraduate education for rural primary care: Strategies for institutional change at New Mexico and Morehouse, *Family Medicine, 15,* 20–24.

CHAPTER 6

Clinical Electives for Preclinical Medical Students

JOAN E. CHRISTY AND ARTHUR KAUFMAN

Renee was awakened by the beeping of the pager on her night table. The illuminated dial of her clock read 1:30 A.M. She called the emergency room at the University Hospital. Dave, an Emergency Room Technician, came to the phone and spoke excitedly, "We've got a 16-year-old rape victim down here. She looks pretty bad—crying and all. The sheriffs are with her. They said she was attacked by about four guys up in the mountains. She was held for hours. Can you come right down?"

Renee was a first-year medical student on call with the rape crisis team composed of volunteer medical, nursing, and pharmacy students. She took a quick look in the mirror and pondered her casual clothing. Maybe the victim would be more comforted seeing someone who looked more professional. She threw on a short white jacket, clipped on her student ID tag, slipped a note pad into her pocket and rushed out the door into the early morning chill.

The Emergency Room was chaotic with doctors and nurses rushing in and out of the trauma rooms trying to stabilize two patients who had been knifed repeatedly in a bar-room brawl. As Dave hurried past, wheeling a stretcher into one of the trauma rooms, he acknowledged Renee with a nod and eyed the corner of the waiting room.

Renee looked over and saw a small form on the last seat in the back row, head down, huddled against the wall. A county sheriff stood beside her with a clipboard, fidgeting with his pen. As Renee approached, the victim looked up at her. She was wrapped in a blanket and was shivering. Mascara streaked down both cheeks, and her left eye was swollen shut.

As Renee sat down, the sheriff demanded to know how long the examination would take—he couldn't hang around all morning. Renee shot up her hand to silence him, not taking her eyes off her young patient. She put her arm around the girl, who dropped magnetically onto Renee's shoulder. Renee asked if she could get her water or anything before she took her back to the examining room. Renee felt in control. She was now able to focus on details— the loose button on her patient's blouse and the tear rolling down the swelling under her right eye.

Goals

1. *Relevance of classroom learning.*   Students should experience, firsthand, the clinical relevance of the basic science coursework they study.
2. *Service while learning.*   Students should be able to offer health care early in their medical education.
3. *Cooperative, early, health care team training.*   Students should be encouraged to work cooperatively with peers and other health science students.
4. *The community, a laboratory for learning.*   The community is as valuable a learning resource as the classroom, hospital, or research bench and should therefore be employed for educational purposes from the beginning of medical school.
5. *Early student exposure to primary care.*   Students should be exposed to primary care practitioners to offer some balance to the almost exclusive exposure to university-based subspecialists.

Introduction

In the seminal experiment at Western Reserve University in the 1950s (Ham, 1962), medical students were assigned to follow a pregnant woman through pregnancy and delivery. Since that time, clinical experiences for beginning medical students have slowly become more common in the preclinical curriculum in many medical schools (Hatch & Lovelace, 1980; Gellhorn & Scheuer, 1978; Spencer, 1980).

These experiences go one step beyond the now-prevalent preclinical behavioral science courses which explore such topics as the physician–patient interaction, human sexuality, the effect of emotional stress on morbidity and mortality, and interviewing techniques. The newer clinical offerings are often focused around a needy community and place preclinical students in a caregiving role with considerable faculty supervision. The student's sense of providing a service while receiving "hands-on" learning can provide a powerful educational incentive. Yet these experiences are criticized by some traditional educators. They view such early clinical endeavors as premature, offered before students have "mastered the basics."

What is the potential contribution of these early, longitudinal experiences in the broad context of preclinical education? Are they especially suited to problem-based programs?

University of New Mexico

The clinical elective program for preclinical medical students at the University of New Mexico was begun in 1975 by the Department of Family and Community Medicine. The program became the wellspring from which many of the underlying principles of PCC were first drawn. It was also the source of our emphases on early clinical content and community-based learning. These distinguish PCC from many of the evolving, problem-based learning experiments worldwide. The clinical electives provided the first vehicle for close interaction between the faculty and the first- and second-year students in clinical settings. Not only did the elective experiences set the stage for the PCC experiment, but they continue to be an integral part of the elective offerings for all students. Clinical electives provide one of the few bridges of interaction between the students in the PCC track and those in the conventional track. The clinical elective program for first- and second-year students has grown from a small effort of one department, to include a variety of elective experiences offered by the majority of clinical departments.

Preparation for the Electives

In 1974, the Department of Family and Community Medicine gave its first lecture-based course for preclinical students, "Introduction to Family and Community Medicine." The course was roundly criticized by the students for its format (once-a-week afternoon lectures) and content. This prodded the Department to examine not only its own strengths and weaknesses, but, perhaps more importantly, its mission in education. As a result, the educational planning group decided that it would be more important to capture the students' imagination, rather than to worry about specific course content. The department also sought to design a course that would capitalize on the "idealism" of new students, a quality which, unfortunately, dwindled rapidly in the environs of conventional medical schools (Rezler, 1974).

The role model that most beginning medical students have in mind is a physician in clinical practice. But the satisfaction of emulating this model by giving care is deferred until the clinical years. Traditionally, preclinical students are usually passive learners, giving nothing to patients and nothing to the community. This can be especially frustrating for the many students who have been committed, active participants in community service prior to entering medical school. Moreover, medical students are trained in isolation from students of other healthcare professions, hindering the development of teamwork skills that are expected to be employed with facility upon graduation (Scher, Ripley, & Johnson, 1975).

With these concerns in mind, the Department embarked upon an experiment designed to supplement the educational environment of preclinical medical students with a longitudinal clinical experience beginning in the first year of medical school. Learning was to be active throughout the experiment. It was believed that if students were active participants in their own education, learning would be optimized. If medical students learned and worked beside nursing and pharmacy students, perhaps they would each learn to share patient-care responsibility. If students were to be with patients, they must also provide a service, not simply observe a doctor–patient interaction. And if students studied sore throats, they must learn the physical examination of the head and neck.

These clinical experiences would, however, be only a small part of the "preclinical" students' curriculum. The department was therefore concerned that the impact of the experiences would be nullified by the pressure and stress of the dominant, basic science coursework. To counteract this effect, a strategy was devised to increase the visibility, acceptability, and impact of the clinical offerings within the school. The Department chose to emphasize the relevance of basic sciences to the problems seen by the practicing physician. This would enhance the students' appreciation for their concurrent, preclinical coursework.

The School of Medicine had long offered several brief courses that introduced first-year students to clinical medicine. Mandatory courses in emergency medicine and clinical interviewing were given during the initial weeks of the first year of school. These were intended to offer an orientation to the study of medicine. However, the skills learned in these courses had no immediate application for the student and were usually forgotten by the time clinical preparation courses appeared, in the second semester of the second year. The Department believed that the addition of a first-term course on the physical diagnosis of common, primary-care problems would give students the knowledge necessary for subsequently providing general health care under close supervision.

But how should the new curricular offering be introduced? Running a "minor" course concurrently with "major" ones like biochemistry or anatomy would dilute the effect of the new course. Therefore, the Department combined all of its course hours into a one-week, solid block of time immediately after final exams in biochemistry and anatomy. The students could now give their undivided attention to the new course. It was called "Primary Care and Its Social Dimensions," and it formed a natural sequence with the brief courses in emergency medicine and clinical interviewing which had been completed a month previously.

The week-long course ran three full days and two half-days (Voorhees et al., 1977). The syllabus contained a potpourri of clinical, basic science, and socioeconomic material organized around common primary-care problems. The material was organized around nine clinical problems: cancer, coronary heart disease, hypertension, peptic ulcer, otitis media, sore throat, alcoholism, smoking, and stress management. For each of the five days, the syllabus included material on physical examination maneuvers, laboratory techniques, case problems (Table 6.1), socioeconomic data, and research articles, all of which the students were to review before the particular day's class.*

Students in the medical school class, and those nursing and pharmacy students planning to take clinical electives subsequently with the medical students, were divided into groups of eight. On Monday, Wednesday, and Friday the groups met in faculty members' homes. The home setting was informal, and it promoted personal exchanges between faculty and students. There they worked on the primary-care problems, practiced the pertinent physical examination maneuvers upon each other, discussed the readings, and worked on the case problems from the syllabus. The Tuesday and Thursday sessions were held in the classrooms, and were devoted to cancer and stress management. In these classroom sessions, the students practiced patient education techniques to reduce stress, reviewed methods of cancer detection, and practiced breast examination on elderly women—volunteers from Rent-A-Granny† (Kaufman, Voorhees, & Suozzi, 1978).

---

*A copy of the 300-page syllabus can be obtained for $10.00 from the Division of Undergraduate Education, Department of Family, Community and Emergency Medicine, 2400 Tucker NE, Albuquerque, NM 87131.

†Rent-A-Granny is a temporary employment service for persons aged 55 or older.

Table 6.1. Case Problem Accompanying Section on Sore Throat

Case III

J. S., a seven-year old boy from a working-class family living in Albuquerque's South Valley, is brought to your office by his mother. She requests that he be treated for strep throat (diagnosed by the New Mexico Heart Association in a "strep culture booth" at a local health fair). He had a sore throat last week when he was cultured, but now feels fine. She also requests that he get his tonsils taken out because he keeps getting "strep throat" and "ear infections."

You take a history and discover that the family consists of nine children and two adults, all living in a five-room, poorly heated, old house.

The father is on social security disability insurance, and the mother does domestic work several times a week.

Questions:

1. Why is there a link between poverty and rheumatic fever?
2. Would you treat the patient now, even though he feels fine?
3. Would you screen the whole family? What are their chances of having strep throat?
4. If you charge the average doctor's fee, how much will it cost to treat this boy? How much to culture his family?
5. Should he have his tonsils out? Defend your answer.

The popularity of the course was overwhelming, and Department faculty felt their stock to be clearly rising among medical students. Faculty who had "bombed" as lecturers the prior year now received rave reviews on (literally) their home turf. They loved working in small, problem-oriented groups. The Department was young and was somewhat insecure in shouldering its two new specialties (family practice and community medicine). Consequently, it was eager to build a supportive constituency within the Medical Center, and this course seemed to present the perfect opportunity. The chairman thus encouraged Department faculty to devote even more contact time with students, which, it was hoped, would generate an even more positive response from the students; and perhaps this response would filter through to the general faculty.

After the students had been introduced to the clinical relevance of basic sciences, and after they had experienced hands-on physical diagnosis and close contact with faculty in the "Primary Care" course, they wanted more action! The Department responded with a series of four half-day, physical examination sessions. This gave more time to practice their newly acquired clinical skills. Even though these sessions were intended for only those students who were interested in immediately applying the skills to a subsequent clinical elective, nearly all of the class members attended. The preclinical students, therefore, by the third month of their first year, felt ready to begin actual clinical contact.

Setting Up the Electives

Over the first two years of the program, ten clinical sites were developed for students choosing to participate in clinical electives. Such sites as corrections facilities and mountain-village storefront clinics were selected because they presented students with obvious health care needs. Thus, students and faculty could couple service with learning. The Department's orientation had always been toward the community. Therefore, faculty involvement in community electives was accepted from the beginning as a legitimate academic function.

Because of time demands, first-year students would be able to offer only a half-day per week for a clinical elective, so sites had to be found either within Albuquerque or within an hour's drive from the University. Further, in order for there to be a stable clinic time for students and patients alike, the existing class schedules would have to be modified. Fortuitously, this pressing need for fixed elective time occurred simultaneously with a move on the part of many faculty and students to reduce the number of classroom hours and to increase independent study time for the students. The School's preclinical curriculum oversight committee responded favorably by establishing Tuesday and Thursday afternoons as free time for preclinical students. The students could use this time for electives or for independent study.

Students would be able to serve at the clinics only once a week, and for only nine months—the school year. There was a question, therefore, regarding whether such a clinic service could really fill a community health care need. And so, at the outset, a goal of the elective was the development of a more permanent kind of health care service at the clinic sites.

Careful planning went into the pursuit of this goal. University representatives held many meetings with those groups in the community who would be directly involved in the utilization of the clinic services. An exciting part of the development of some of the electives was the central role that the health science students played in negotiating the terms of service. They confronted the community concerns personally and decided upon the types of services that would be offered. The students who set up a clinic at a prison honor farm had to convince prison administrators that women students would be safe from sexual advances of male inmates. They ran a literature search and found that the level of violence in prisons actually diminishes when prisons are staffed with men and women alike. Students who set up a sexual-assault response team, in the county hospital, worked with the community-based Rape Crisis Center to allay fears that the latter's already established services would be undermined.

To pay for the books, equipment, and travel that could not be funded in other ways, most students in the electives volunteered to work for two or three days during their summer break, screening 600 children for a University-sponsored summer sports program. The screening, supervised by faculty, earned the elective program $2,000 each year to cover these costs.

There was a concern about the medical school's legal responsibility for the services provided by students at the clinics. But the University lawyer stated that the students' activities, while in the community, were covered by the University faculty malpractice insurance.

By the end of the first two years of the elective program, 63 percent of the preclinical medical students had participated in the electives. Each of these students served at one of the ten sites for a minimum of one academic year. Offerings in the 1975–1976 academic year are presented in Table 6.2.

Table 6.2.   Electives during 1975–1976

Elective	Medical Students	Nursing and Pharmacy Students
Rape-crisis and follow-up care	10	2
Prison health care	8	5
Nursing home clinic	8	4
Home health care	10	—
Rural Clinic #1	2	—
Rural Clinic #2	7	2
Rescue mission	3	—
Children's shelter clinic	4	2
Patient support service	2	—
Death and dying/hospice care	4	—
	58	15

The populations that are served by the clinical electives are diverse in socioeconomic levels, lifestyles, and special health care needs. The ten elective sites presently in operation can be divided into four categories: institutional health care, care for the aged, crisis intervention and care, and other care modalities.

Case Example

Selecting and developing these elective sites has been as much a function of responding to community needs as it has been one of supporting students in their community-oriented efforts. The students' sense of responsibility to their clinical duties has resulted, not only in enhancement of student learning, but also in improved health-care delivery to the community itself. A brief case history of one elective, the prison honor farm, is illustrative (Kaufman et al., 1979).

In 1975, a group of students toured the Los Lunas Honor Farm, a small, minimum-security prison, 30 miles south of Albuquerque, housing 200 inmates. The center had no on-site medical facilities, and so students selected it as the setting of their longitudinal elective clinical experience. Inmates requiring emergency care had been referred to the closest hospital emergency room, 19 miles away, or to the infirmary at the State Penitentiary in Santa Fe, 90 miles away. It was the responsibility of administrators and guards to judge the validity and severity of the inmates' medical complaints and make appropriate referrals. Because of the inconvenience and expense of transportation, "minor" ailments were often neglected until they became "major." But a fear of subsequent legal suits was pervasive among prison administrators. Consequently, they were very glad to have a clinic on the premises.

In consultation with the students, the prison administration invested $1,500 to convert an abandoned fruit cannery on the grounds into a small clinic. The inmates proudly constructed and decorated their new facility. It had four examining rooms, a laboratory area, and a waiting room. The first student health team consisted of eight preclinical medical students, four senior nursing students, and two senior pharmacy students. They were supervised by two faculty members, one from the Department of Family and Community Medicine, and the other from the College of Nursing. During its first year, the clinic was operated one afternoon a week.

The clinic originally opened on a walk-in basis, but soon had to convert to an appointment system when over 20 patients appeared weekly for service. Patients came on their own initiative, both for general physical checkups and for acute problems, the vast majority being in the latter category. Students interviewed patients and performed physical examinations. Their findings and management plans were reviewed by the faculty members.

Student reaction to the Honor Farm experience has been consistently positive. Their work has had a great impact on their attitudes toward prison health as a practice choice, toward health care for prisoners in general, and toward the relevancy of their regular curricular course work.

> *"I was initially afraid, but now I see them [the inmates] just as other individuals."*

> *"They really have a dire need for general medical care on a regular, nonthreatening basis."*

> *"My big problem in studying for medical school seems to be the lack of relevance. This experience gave me at least a good reason to study. It told me that you actually need to know some of the basic sciences."*

At the outset, prison staff members had reservations about voluntary student medical help. They feared that students might be "conned" by the inmates, or that the students might become entangled in the inmates' nonmedical problems. They were also afraid that student participation would be episodic—with a large student turnover. Over the years, none of these fears has materialized, and a mutual trust and respect has developed among the students, staff, and inmates.

The success of the Honor Farm experience stimulated interest on the part of the State Penitentiary Warden in remedying deficiencies of health care services in other system facilities. At that time, the penitentiary population of 1,200 men and 40 women was served by only a part-time surgeon and four technicians. The warden realized that, with such understaffing, the medical needs at the facility were not being met. He approached the University's Department of Family, Community and Emergency Medicine for assistance.

The result was a joint recruitment effort, by the University and Department of Corrections, which led to the hiring of a full-time prison physician. He was designated as the Medical Director of the Division of Corrections and was appointed as a clinical associate professor within the Department of Family, Community and Emergency Medicine. He reorganized the health services in all the state prison facilities and added a full-time nurse practitioner at the Honor Farm and several physician's assistants at the main penitentiary. The result has been a far more integrated, higher quality medical care system for the inmates of the state correction facilities. Because of these changes, the need for student services at the Honor Farm has diminished, but a scaled-down student elective program still exists. Ironically, the success of the elective has reduced its necessity. This may be the ideal result for such University outreach projects. If a university is to conserve its resources for the broadest possible community service, then each project should determine means by which the recipient community or agency can attract permanent, professional service apart from the University.

Modifications of Electives for PCC Students

Initially, the introduction of the Primary Care Curriculum (PCC) had little effect on the elective program from which it had sprung. Clinical electives were required of PCC students in preparation for their extended rural preceptorships offered at the end of the first year of school. As in all elective offerings, the experiences were not standardized, and students' skills were unassessed. As a consequence, when PCC students in the first two classes entered their rural sites, many found that their clinical skills were inadequate. PCC planners increasingly realized the importance of clinical skills and the competency later expected at rural sites. It was clear that the electives for PCC students could not continue to be "free form" experiences, but must become settings in which clinical skills were monitored and enhanced.

Electives for First-Year Students

In order to correlate the clinical electives more closely with the rural rotations, specific goals were developed for the students in the electives. The preceptors were then provided with a more extensive orientation to the PCC curricular method and to the more guiding roles they were now expected to play in the students' learning. They were asked to allow their students increasing interaction with patients and to provide a specific time during which students could present patients and discuss the patients' problems. The preceptors were also asked to observe and to provide immediate feedback on the students' techniques and effectiveness. This was to be done on at least two occasions for each student. Despite the increased demands on their time, most preceptors welcomed the new guidelines. They felt that the clear expectations added purpose to their work with the students and involved preceptors more responsibly in the educational process.

Electives for Second-Year Students

The demands for elective experiences by second-year students are very different from those of first-year students. Students returning from their extended rural preceptorships, at the conclusion of their first year, bring with them a new clarity of purpose and a better definition of needs.

> *"Hey, they do a lot of surgery out there! . . . I've got to learn more about routine procedures."*

> *"I didn't get much exposure to obstetrics. . . . I'd like to work on that for a while and then switch to . . ."*

Electives planners for Phase II students are sensitive to students' changing needs. These students soon will be starting in-hospital clinical clerkships and rotations. As the reality of this next step takes hold, the students begin to experience anxiety over their ability to function effectively on the in-hospital wards.

Institutionalization and
Impact of Electives

At the University of New Mexico, the popularity of the electives has led to institution-wide expansion of the program. It is now administered by the Office of Undergraduate Medical Education, and the catalog has elective offerings from many departments.*

The impact of the electives is being realized at the residency level as well. The popularity of the electives among students and faculty has led to a longitudinal, community-based program within the Family Practice residency. Currently, all second- and third-year residents select a community clinic site at which they provide service one-half day per week. Almost all of these locations are also student elective sites. The participation of the residents, therefore, further expands and professionalizes the services of the community health care teams. In addition, the increased interaction between the residents and preclinical students enhances the educational benefit to both.

Problems. Although the elective program has grown into an accepted, integral part of the preclinical curriculum for students in both the PCC and conventional tracks, many problems remain. The program is the only continuous educational experience that brings the students of both tracks together. While the electives are required of PCC students, they are optional for conventional-track students. Furthermore, PCC students must participate in the more clinical, hands-on electives. Since these tend to be the more popular offerings, conventional-track students often complain of having less access to these electives than do the PCC

---

*A copy of the Electives Program Catalog can be obtained by writing to the Office of Undergraduate Medical Education, School of Medicine, University of New Mexico, Albuquerque, NM 87131.

students. PCC therefore must be careful to include students from both tracks in these particular electives.

One of the initial interests of the faculty who were establishing the electives was to orient students toward community health needs. But the focus on community dimensions of the electives has been superseded in many cases by the goal of helping students refine their clinical skills. Program planners are concerned that the shift has been too great and are exploring ways of properly balancing the emphasis.

Another shift that concerns PCC planners is the change in outlook that occurs among students as they make the transition from the first to the second preclinical year. Second-year students seem more pressured by anxiety about their upcoming National Boards. For these students, a conflict emerges between using nontutorial time for clinical electives or for Board study. A number of students worry about the approaching, in-hospital clinical rotations in their third year and try to prepare by spending this second year rotating among a number of specialist preceptors. Because of such a wide diversity of student needs, it is extremely difficult for PCC to plan this portion of the program effectively. A great deal of flexibility and time are required of the program coordinators, who often feel that they are involved in an administrative nightmare. One remedy gaining increasing popularity is for house officers who have graduated from PCC to serve as in-hospital preceptors for second-year PCC students. This builds a student/graduate network, and reduces the faculty teaching loads.

Over the years, the relative popularity of the various clinical electives has changed, reflecting shifting national interests. For example, the needs of sexual assault victims were emerging in the national consciousness in the late 1970s, and the Sexual Assault Response Team elective attracted the largest number of participants. But as care for sexual assault victims entered the mainstream of medicine, the novelty of such service waned, and student enthusiasm for the elective diminished. The electives that are now gaining in popularity are those that reflect the newer national interest in physical fitness, sports medicine, and emergency medicine. The pressure on the clinical elective faculty to keep pace with shifting student interests can create a heavy administrative burden. New activities have to be developed, and old ones, at times, phased out.

Lessons Learned

1. Curriculum planners should seek fixed, weekly "free time" or "elective time" within the preclinical curriculum.

2. The teaching of clinical skills should be instituted early in the medical students' first year.
3. To broaden the base of support for such a program within the school, faculty from different clinical departments should be recruited to participate from the beginning of a clinical electives program.
4. Community elective sites should be selected at which students can offer a needed service.
5. The community-based clinical electives should serve as a vehicle to foster an alliance among students in different health science programs (e.g., medicine, nursing, and pharmacy).
6. The academic legitimacy of a community-based, clinical elective program should be promoted among faculty to encourage their support.

Experience at Other Schools

The Commitment to the Underserved People (CUP) program at the University of Arizona is a student-run, co-curricular elective spanning four years of medical school (Spencer & Outcalt, 1980). The program was developed in response to (1) the needs of large, underserved segments of the population, and (2) first-year medical student idealism, which is increasingly frustrated over the course of formal study.

In 1978, the College of Medicine held a seminar on underserved people, after which participating students obtained faculty support for a longitudinal program involving students in hands-on care for the underserved. The Department of Family and Community Medicine became the base for this effort, though faculty from other primary-care departments and from the community now participate.

Each year, between 12 and 20 first-year students choose to join the CUP program. The only grossly discernible difference between CUP and nonparticipating students is found in program preference by sex. While 35 percent of each admitted class are women, 50 percent of students electing CUP are women (perhaps an important parallel with the percentage of women selecting the University of New Mexico's PCC Program).

CUP focuses upon three areas of concern—curriculum, service, and support (Pust & Moher, 1983):

1. *CUP curriculum.* CUP students are encouraged to take noncredit, community-based electives, throughout their

four years and summer rotations, in communities where underserved populations predominate. In addition, in a course segment entitled Department of Family and Community Medicine Preparation for Clinical Medicine, CUP students are grouped into tutorials in which case-based, problem-solving discussions, led by CUP faculty, are presented from the perspective of the physician in an underserved area.

2. *Service while studying.* In the first semester, students visit six to ten Tucson facilities (e.g., church-run clinics, Indian clinics, hospices) which serve the poor. In the second and third semester, each student chooses one of these sites and provides care there one-half day per week. The students themselves have initiated a number of new clinic services. Since 1980, a weekly clinic, in the community of Dar a Luz, has provided prenatal care to a weekly average of 20 Hispanic, low-income women. Other CUP students have organized a Saturday clinic in South Tucson.

3. *Emphasis of program.* The CUP Program emphasizes the three classically underserved groups: inner-city minorities, scattered rural populations, and Third World countries. Arizona is 80 percent urban; it is lacking in mid-size cities, and thus its rural population is isolated; it is situated on a Third World (Mexican) border. Thus, the three groups form a natural mission for Arizona's CUP Program. There is special emphasis on International Health, and on the two-way transfer of learning that occurs between the experiences of those working with the domestic underserved and those with the Third World groups.

The CUP model is one that can be introduced into a totally conventional medical school, requiring no curricular modifications. Yet the program can sustain the interests of the community-oriented segment of the student body and can develop important service links between the medical school and the needier portions of its surrounding community. The Director, Dr. Ron Pust, has said,

"The program keeps students from becoming submerged in formal medical school to the point of forgetting their commitment. The focus is on the total needs of the community. The whole world is out there, if we will but remain part of it." (Personal communication, 1984)

Implications

Community-based clinical electives provide a nurturing environment for experimental approaches to medical education. The sites are often physically remote from the mother institution, the situations place the students in direct contact with real-life problems, and the students work in small groups in which faculty–student interaction is more personal and supportive than at the medical center. In fact, many clinical elective programs are clear examples of community-oriented, problem-based learning and can become the impetus for broader changes in a similar vein within the conventional curriculum.

Experience has demonstrated that preclinical students not only can function as responsible, adult learners but also can be useful health care providers early in their education if given adequate preparation, and supervision, by medical school faculty. Experiences like those illustrated enhance the outreach of the medical school and increase its positive profile in the community. The elective experiences can have important effects on the processes of institutional and educational change, because of the impact of the experience on the students, the medical school, and the community.

Through the electives, students can find increased relevance in their basic science curriculum, as well as a broader perspective on the relationship between a patient's health problems, lifestyle, and environment. Students from medicine, nursing, and pharmacy work cooperatively on a health service project and gain important team skills not taught in a conventional curriculum. As health care delivery systems are becoming increasingly complex and interdependent, effective teamwork is becoming absolutely essential.

In addition to benefiting students and patients, community experiences can also provide a fertile clinical base for the research, service, and education requirements of the faculty. Far from diverting faculty time from useful research, clinical electives themselves have the potential for enhancing academic productivity.

References

Geiger, J. H. (1980, Jan.–Feb.). Sophie Davis School of Education at City College of New York prepares primary care physicians for practice in underserved inner-city areas. *Public Health Reports, 95,* 32–37.

Gellhorn, A., & Scheuer, R. (1978). The experiment in medical education at the City College of New York. *Journal of Medical Education, 53,* 574–582.

Ham, T. H. (1962). Medical education at Western Reserve University: A progress report for the sixteen years, 1946–1962. *New England Journal of Medicine, 267,* 868–874.

Hatch, J. W., & Lovelace, K. A. (1980, Jan.–Feb.). Involving the Southern rural church and students of the health professions in health education. *Public Health Reports, 95,* 23–25.

Kaufman, A., Holbrook, J., Collier, I., Farabough, J., Jackson, R., & Johnston, T. (1979). Prison health and medical education. *Journal of Medical Education, 54,* 925–931.

Kaufman, A., Voorhees, D., & Suozzi, P. (1978). Senior citizens as live breast examination models. *Journal of Medical Education, 53,* 997.

Pust, R. F., & Moher, L. M. (1983). Promoting medical careers in underserved areas. *Arizona Medicine, 40,* 397–401.

Rezler, A. G. (1974). Attitude changes during medical school: a review of the literature. *Journal of Medical Education, 49,* 1023.

Scher, M. E., Ripley, H. S., & Johnson, M. H. (1975). Stereotyping and role conflicts between medical students and psychiatric nurses. *Hospital Community Psychiatry, 26,* 219.

Spencer, S. S., & Outcalt, D. (1980, Jan.–Feb.) Commitment to Underserved People (CUP) Program at the University of Arizona. *Public Health Reports, 95,* 26–28.

Voorhees, J. D., Kaufman, A., Heffron, W., Jackson, R., DiVasto, P., Wiese, W., & Daitz, B. (1977). Teaching preclinical medical students in a clinical setting. *Journal of Family Practice, 5,* 464–465.

Extended Community Preceptorship: Problem-Based Learning in the Field

J. DAYTON VOORHEES, MAX D. BENNETT,
AND ALEKSANDRA COUNSELLOR

Hi! Sorry I missed you. My rural rotation is going great—I love it! I've been taking care of an "undocumented worker," 29 years old, with a full-blown case of tetanus. It's been good practice using my Spanish also! We had him on Pavulon, did a tracheostomy yesterday and now he's doing okay—just on Valium (lots!). In fact, so much the Roche rep called the hospital to see what was going on! I think he's enough of a fighter that he'll pull through. There's a mad dash to get a booster these days in Silver City. Take care!

Amy

The note was from a first year PCC student during her extended rural clerkship in Silver City, a small, southwestern New Mexico town hard hit by unemployment after the closing of the local copper mine. Amy was experiencing the joy of learning and caring for patients, taking greater responsibility for her education, and learning a breadth of health issues experientially. She would be able to balance her upcoming clinical clerkships in our university hospital with an appreciation for the excitement and complexity of primary care in a rural community.

Goals

1. *To provide students with a better balance of clinical experiences reflecting the world of practice.* The students' traditional tertiary-care, specialty-based hospital clerkships should be complemented by a sustained, community-based, primary-care experience to expose students to the variety, complexity, and opportunities for medical practice.

2. *To provide students with a community "laboratory" for applying problem-based learning skills gained at the university.* Students should undergo sustained, real-life experiences integrating the clinical reasoning process and self-motivated study with patient care. The field experience should help the student to transfer problem-based learning skills from tutorial groups on campus to individual study in the community.

3. *To provide students with a real-life context for learning relevant social sciences.* The community offers a natural setting for learning and applying knowledge in such important (but traditionally underemphasized) subjects as epidemiology, community and public health, sociology, and health economics. Such knowledge enables students to gain skills in assessing the demographic, community dimensions of health problems.

4. *To gain skills in working effectively with other health professionals and community representatives.* The field experience should reinforce the concept that the physician is but one component of a health care team, each of whose differently trained members is a vital resource to the community's health. Effective coordination between members of the team should be seen as a necessity for optimum community health care services.

Introduction

Clinical, problem-based learning in the classroom, with its heavy reliance on written and acted simulations, inevitably leads to a desire on the part of students to take the next step, to experience the real-life application of this knowledge. While clinical electives or week-ly visits to community health care sites in the preclinical years provide some satisfaction of this need, students profit even more from a sus-tained immersion in real-life, problem-based learning by means of community-based preceptorships.

Preceptorships have played a steadily increasing role in medical education. They have been seen as a means of counterbalancing the subspecialty emphasis that was experienced by students at their univer-sity medical centers. It was hoped the preceptors might entice students to enter primary-care careers in rural or underserved areas. However, whereas most studies show that specialty choice decisions are made during the third year of medical school (Harris & Elbert, 1983; Paiva, 1982; Quenck & Smith, 1976), most preceptorships are offered in the fourth year. At best, fourth-year preceptorships support already es-tablished career-choice and practice-site preferences. They offer too little too late.

A concern emerging in the past decade, extends beyond the spe-cialty and geographic choices made by physicians. It is related to the choices they make regarding the extent of their roles in their chosen communities (Mullan, 1982). If the physician of the future is to foster preventive services in this practice community, where will he learn the requisite skills in epidemiology, health economics, medical anthropolo-gy, and environmental risk analysis? One educator commented, "Learn-ing primary care medicine in a university is like trying to learn forestry in a lumberyard" (Verby, Schaefer, & Voeks, 1981). The dominance of the tertiary care training center in the clinical education of medical students crowds out such important community-oriented concerns.

University of New Mexico Program

Compared to most preceptorships offered in medical educa-tion, the phase IB preceptorship of the Primary Care Curriculum pro-gram is unique in three characteristics:

1. Placement in the curriculum—during the first year, after six and one-half months of medical school.
2. Length—a required 16 weeks.
3. Educational philosophy—student-centered and problem-based.

During the preceptorship, students are matched with practicing primary-care physicians throughout New Mexico and remain affiliated with one site for the duration of this phase. Preceptors care for a variety of patient populations representing the cultural diversity of New Mexico and its varied patterns of medical practice. Locations range from a Navajo Community Clinic to a private group practice in an old Spanish village, representing the cultural, economic, and ethnic diversity of the state (Figure 7.1). Sites are located as far as 300 miles from the medical school. Phase IB is carefully designed to build on the problem-solving,

Figure 7.1.   Map of New Mexico with local features of Phase IB preceptorship sites.

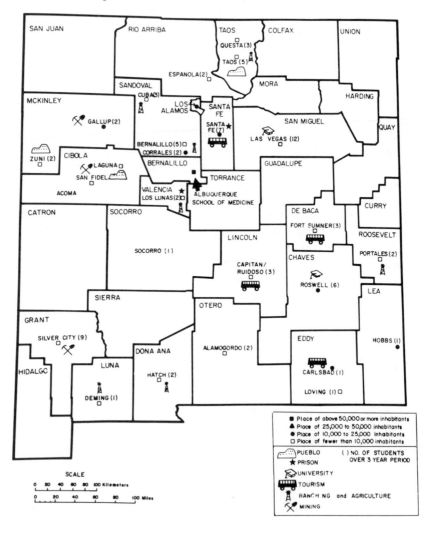

clinical, and resource-identification skills students have gained in Phase IA. It allows students the opportunity to refine their problem-based learning skills and transfer them to a clinical setting in a small community. The students' primary focus during this phase is the independent learning of basic and clinical science based on patient problems derived from the preceptor's practice and community. Seen within the context of the entire PCC curriculum, Phase IB is notable for the following features:

1. Movement from group to independent learning.
2. Use of actual patients and their problems on a daily basis as a springboard for the study of the sciences basic to medicine.
3. Opportunity to be introduced to the elements of community medicine and to view medicine from a community perspective.
4. Firsthand experience with the impact of being a physician on one's personal life and lifestyle.

The mechanics of Phase IB can be broken into elements and considered individually.

Preceptorship and Site Selection

Each student is assigned to a principal preceptor who is a primary-care physician (family practice, internal medicine, or pediatrics). The preceptor is responsible for supervising the entire Phase IB experience and is primarily responsible for evaluating the student. Since a student spends a portion of almost every day with the principal preceptor over a 16-week period, the faculty role of the preceptor is more intense and more personal than the role most traditional medical school faculty members play in either preclinical or clinical years. Thus, preceptor selection must be conducted carefully.

Characteristics used to evaluate potential preceptors include such areas as competence in the practice of medicine; philosophical support of the PCC program and its nontraditional approach to medical education; and willingness and ability to take an average of about one-half to one hour per day to interact with the student.

The pool of potential preceptors was initially culled from the preceptors for the existing fourth-year preceptorship offered by the School of Medicine. This provided an important screening mechanism, for in many cases there were years of senior-student feedback on potential preceptors. Currently, each practice is visited and evaluated by a PCC faculty member. Students from the previous year's Phase IB are also asked to evaluate their preceptors. Prospective Phase IB students are then given a list of approved preceptors, and a "matching" process begins. The students visit the sites they find appealing. Then they submit a list of those sites in order of preference. The preceptors, in turn, are consulted about their preference of students. The Phase IB coordinator uses this information to determine the best possible match.

The success of this effort is reflected in the high regard in which the selected preceptors have been held by the students. Typical comments follow:

> *"[He was a] preceptor with time to spend with me reviewing the material I covered. . . . I had a feeling of freedom to set up the type of experience I was comfortable with. Other physicians in town were willing to take time for me. . . . [I appreciated the] openness of the hospital staff and their cooperation with my education."*

> *"My preceptor talked to me a lot about his experiences being a Hispanic medical student, of having been raised on a farm and all the pressures he experiences being a doctor in his home town. He is still considered a young boy by many people in the community. He has helped me think about different aspects of returning home to practice."*

Preceptor Education

Each year a two-day workshop is held prior to Phase IB at the medical school for preceptors, students, and supervising faculty. The workshop covers the philosophy and educational methods of PCC and the goals of Phase IB. In the workshop, each student and his or her preceptor develop specific goals and objectives for the student's upcoming experience. The workshop has proven to be an important transitional step for preceptors, who must now bridge the gap between their own, traditional medical school instruction and their students' problem-based education. Continuing medical education credits are available to the preceptors for attending the workshop.

Format of Phase IB

A student generally spends half of his or her time in a patient-care setting and half in independent study. About 10 to 15 patients are usually seen per week per student, but there is wide variation because of the different abilities and interests of the students and the character of the physician's practice.

After adjusting to the clinic routine, students usually take histories and perform physical examinations, and then present their findings to the preceptor, who reviews the student's work. Students become involved in the management of the patient problems, but their primary focus is to derive basic and clinical science learning issues from the patient problems, which are then used as springboards for independent study. Each student is encouraged to develop a personal system of recording patient encounters and learning issues.

Educational Support System

Students are able to obtain materials from the Medical Center Library quickly and efficiently (Chapter 4). A single staff member in the library is identified as the liaison person, and Phase IB students can receive journal articles, books, literature searches, and audiovisual programs, usually within 24 hours. Funds are also available for long distance calls from the preceptorship sites to faculty at the UNM School of Medicine for consultation. The message to the student is that rural practice does not necessarily entail a lack of access to professional resources.

University-based faculty members serve as "circuit riders," each of whom visits one to three sites every two to four weeks. By reviewing the students' progress and observing the interactions between students and preceptors, circuit riders play a major role in organizing, evaluating, and providing moral support for participants during the Phase IB experience. Circuit riders also serve as a personal link between the School of Medicine faculty, the students, and the preceptors.

Students take their own books, journal articles, and other resources to the Phase IB site. By setting up their own information systems and reviewing those used by the preceptors, most students can learn the long-term importance of careful cataloguing of new knowledge and information.

Community Medicine Aspects

In addition to learning about the sciences basic to medicine, students experience what it is like to be a medical provider in a nonurban area, to become a part of the community, and to pursue community medicine learning issues.

To facilitate the introduction of the student into the community, many techniques are employed. Community newspapers may run introductory articles, the preceptor may ask the student to make a case presentation to the hospital staff, or the student may be asked to speak to the local Rotary Club or Kiwanis. Often preceptors have been active in such community service organizations, and students learn the preeminent social role in which physicians may be placed in smaller communities. Students also observe the time and social pressures on a physician in a small community. Thus, the students observe in a very personal way how different preceptors combine their professional, family, and personal activities. It is impossible to predict how students will react to a particular preceptor's practice pattern, community involvement, or lifestyle. PCC can only encourage students to keep an open mind and learn from positive and negative experiences. It is important that students not become "appendages" or "apprentices" to the preceptor, but remain critical observers, always learning.

"Community-oriented primary care" is a new term which denotes the philosophical orientation of Phase IB. It implies that primary care services include an appraisal of the health status of a group of individuals or families in the community, a plan for needed intervention, then evaluation of the effects of the intervention (Mullan, 1982). A major educational goal for Phase IB therefore is to provide students with a community experience that will allow an understanding of how community problems affect groups as well as individuals. For example, one student noted symptoms of depression in a copper miner who had been laid off. She did a community survey on the families of the town's unemployed and found a sharp rise in reported cases of wife beating, child abuse, and marital discord. To introduce students to this community approach, they are given a week-long introduction to community medicine during Phase IA. The problems highlight community medicine issues, and the tutors are drawn from the Division of Community Medicine.

While at their IB sites, students are required to complete one of three community medicine research or service options:

1. Students briefly investigate five issues. An example of one issue is: Identify two patients whose illnesses were caused by the environment (work place, home, or general community environment). What did you do to help prevent these problems from affecting other people in the same environment?

2. Identify, investigate, analyze, and write a report about *one* community medicine topic which you investigate in more depth than what is expected in option 1 above. The topic should involve a health problem within the community or within an identifiable population of the community (such as diabetics, farm laborers, or people afflicted with shigella).

3. A community service project may be pursued by students. The project must be in the health area and must meet a need of the

community. Examples include teaching a cardiopulmonary resuscitation class in the high schools and establishing pre-natal classes for indigent, high-risk mothers.

Administration and Finances

Because the preceptorship sites are scattered throughout New Mexico, the fifth largest state geographically, the administration of the program is logistically complex. When a problem arises in a remote site, the distances from the School of Medicine complicate both identification and solution of the problem. For example, one student in a remote site was not being given sufficient patient contact nor adequate supervision by her preceptor. The problem came to light four weeks into Phase IB during the circuit rider's second visit to the community. Recommendations for improvement were made to the student and preceptor, but by the third visit, six weeks into IB, insufficient progress on the problem had been made and new preceptors in the community were enlisted into the program.

Preceptors are not paid for participation in Phase IB and this has both positive and negative aspects. On the positive side, it serves to select physicians who are more dedicated to an educational idea, helps keep costs down, and makes the program more palatable to state legislators, who might balk at providing state funding for private physicians. On the negative side, it means that the program has little contractual hold on the preceptor in terms of making certain that program obligations are met. As partial compensation, preceptors are given several indirect benefits:

1. Clinical appointments to their respective department.
2. Travel and per diem reimbursement for attending the educational workshop.
3. Facilitated medical center library service during preceptorship.

The 17-page curriculum for Phase IB covers the major goals and evaluation methods.* Included are suggestions about time allocation, practical ways to achieve goals, and a format for students and preceptors to address basic and clinical science objectives.

*A copy of the Phase IB curriculum document may be obtained by writing to: Aleksandra Counsellor, M.S., Department of Family, Community and Emergency Medicine, Preceptorship Office, University of New Mexico School of Medicine, Albuquerque, New Mexico 87131.

The budget for Phase IB for 1983 was approximately $2,500 per student (Figure 7.2). The largest portion, one-third, was budgeted for housing and utility expenses for the students. Most students have not been able to discontinue their housing obligations in Albuquerque while they have been at the Phase IB sites and consequently have had to maintain two housing units. Because of the long distances in New Mexico, preceptor sites have been selected in clusters to hold down the travel expenses and time commitments for circuit riders.

No faculty salaries are included in Phase IB PCC budget. Two faculty members are responsible for the preceptorship, and the portion of their salaries attributable to PCC are contributed by their departments.

Results

Five classes, totaling 84 students, have now completed the Phase IB experience of the PCC program. One can draw preliminary conclusions regarding the effects of this program on preceptors and students and on the relationships between the University's medical center and the practice communities.

Preceptors. Fifty-six physicians have participated as primary preceptors (65% family physicians; 35% internists and pediatricians) while an additional 92 have participated as secondary preceptors (including surgeons, pathologists, and radiologists). The latter devote considerable time to the students' education but are not responsible for evaluating or coordinating activities for the student or maintaining a liaison with the medical school. Types of preceptor practice are listed in Table 7.1.

Almost all of the physicians who have served as preceptors have asked to be included as preceptors on a continuing basis. Two physicians

Table 7.1.   Type of Practice for 56 Primary Preceptors

Private practice		
Solo	12	(21%)
Group	21	(38%)
Indian Health Service	7	(13%)
Community clinic	8	(14%)
National Health Service Corps	8	(14%)

Figure 7.2. PCC Phase IB budget: $50,500.

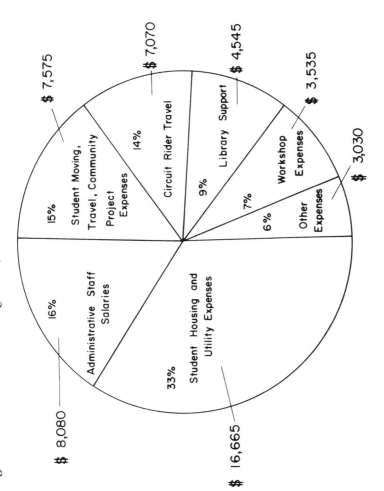

have been replaced by the program while in the midst of the preceptor-ship. The program felt one preceptor had an inappropriate attitude toward the program, the student, and medical education in general. In the second instance, the preceptor was judged to be too busy to spend the necessary time with the student. One of the few students removed from her first site described her frustration: "It was hard trying to explain and prove the worth of PCC to the first preceptor. He did not understand that a time commitment to a PCC student was greater than that to a fourth-year student."

PCC represents a significantly different form of medical education than that experienced by the preceptors during their own medical school careers. As a result, despite a willingness to participate in the program, there often exists considerable skepticism among preceptors during their initial exposure to the program.

One concern in the planning stages of IB was that the combination of the length of the preceptorship, together with the beginning educational level of the students would present too much of a burden on the preceptors. However, when the preceptors were asked to rate their level of enthusiasm at the end of the preceptorships compared to the beginning, 65 percent felt equal or greater enthusiasm for the program at the end. Others were still enthusiastic about the program but more sober about the considerable time demands on their practice.

Results from a two-year survey (1980–1981) of 30 preceptors' responses to carefully selected questions designed to measure their assessment of the effect the preceptorship had upon the day-to-day functioning of their practice are summarized in Table 7.2. Participation resulted in longer hours for a significant percentage of preceptors. It also required them to alter their usual work routines. This usually took place in the area of scheduling, lunch time, and an extension of their work day. These were burdens which fell mainly to the preceptor and were not shared by the preceptor's staff.

Even though the preceptors were not paid and they usually ex-perienced an increased work load, the rewards of participation were great enough to motivate almost all of the preceptors to request continu-ing participation. They found the intellectual stimulation to be signifi-cant, and the students' contribution to actual medical care was very important. There was also a spill-over of benefits to the preceptors' clinic staffs. On many occasions, the staff members felt educationally enriched by the presence of the students. Students often prepared in-formal conferences and teaching materials for the staff. For example, one student conducted topical discussions on such subjects as diabetes

Table 7.2. Preceptors' Perception of the Effect of Phase IB PCC Students on Their Practice

	Preceptor Response by % N=30				
	Strongly Agree	Agree	No Opinion	Disagree	Strongly Disagree
1. Extended your office hours	0	44.8	6.9	34.5	13.8
2. Disrupted the normal flow of work	0	44.8	3.4	34.5	17.2
3. Increased your work load	3.4	58.6	0	38.0	0
4. Increased your staff work load	0	31.0	6.9	62.1	0
5. Provided intellectual stimulation for you	41.4	55.2	3.4	0	0
6. Student interacted with staff educationally	37.5	58.3	0	4.2	0
7. Contributed to medical care of patient in a way that would not have happened otherwise	3.4	58.6	6.9	31.0	0

and hypertension. Another obtained preserved brains for dissection and neuroanatomic discussions for the local nursing school. Many preceptors felt that the presence of a student contributed to the medical care of the patients in ways that may not have occurred had the student not been present. For example, one student helped computerize his preceptor's medical records. Another set up a low-back-pain clinic for his preceptor's patients, and a third translated for the preceptor's Spanish-speaking patients and did home visit follow-ups.

One reason this type of experience is so acceptable to the preceptors relates directly to the educational goals of the phase. Although traditional fourth-year preceptorship students may see a larger number of patients, Phase IB students spend only half of their time in the office, and see but one to three patients, using the contact primarily as a springboard into independent study. Frequently the patient may be hospitalized so that the student–patient encounter takes place outside the clinic. Thus, the preceptor is not burdened by having a student constantly over his or her shoulder, tying up examining rooms, and interfering with the efficient operation of the office.

For physicians who practice in the rural communities of New Mexico and did not train at its university, there is little opportunity to establish a comfortable, working relationship with medical school faculty. However, 66 percent of preceptors felt that their participation in the program enabled them to develop just such ties. Sixty-five percent of the preceptors felt that their communities have directly benefited from the program.

Students. For most students the IB preceptorship has been an outstanding feature of their medical school experience. Twenty-four percent of the students have extended their preceptorships beyond the required 16 weeks, thus forgoing some of their vacation. The intensity of the experience is unexpected for many. Being the sole student at a site, and having the preceptor, office staff, and community people competing for his or her attention often engenders strong feelings of self-worth.

By spending such an extended period of time in this type of setting, students are afforded a realistic view of the responsibilities, requirements, advantages, and disadvantages of rural primary care. For most, this has resulted in a reinforcement of previously held desires to choose this sort of career. One student wrote,

> "I'm looking forward to it more now than ever. Patients are more enjoyable than I thought previously. I'm also beginning to see ways in which I might be able to change some of the more archaic philosophies of the medical community relevant to teaching and interaction among peers, at least in my own immediate environment. I'm definitely committed to primary care now."

Students were asked to consider how their preceptors integrated medicine with family and personal life, and to reflect upon how medicine might interrelate with the important elements in their own lives.

> "I was fortunate to see three different styles of practice. Dr. F. had made the conscious decision to dedicate very nearly his entire life to medicine, and apparently has few regrets. Dr. G. loves his work,

but, in my opinion, is a veritable slave to his profession. And, finally, Dr. T. has consciously determined that his personal and family life take high priority and that he will make time for his family, even if at the cost of time/attention to patients. He is an excellent physician, as are all three, but I feel gratified to have been able to see that one can play some role in determining how one's professional and personal life balance out."

"There is a side to medicine which must have the greatest precision. There is also a very human quality that can't be overlooked. I think I gained as much observing Dr. D. talking with people, hugging the little old ladies, laughing at the comments they often made to him, as I ever did in a basic science lecture."

As some students learn more about primary-care medicine, they realize that they should consider other specialties. A number of students, for example, have discovered they would not function well in a small town.

"I am more aware of the hazards of a small-town practice—the stress of constant call, the gossip of small town and the social position of the doctor."

Other students developed a more sober attitude toward the stresses of practice in general.

"During my preceptorship I saw many physicians who have been divorced . . . spending so much time with physicians forced me to consider the strain which is placed on family relationships by the profession. I have had some rather in-depth conversations about it with my fiancee."

Phase IB thus provides students with a more realistic basis upon which to plan the rest of their elective medical school experiences.

Students have overwhelmingly felt that their preceptorship experience has underscored the need to understand basic sciences. Forty-seven percent strongly agreed and 44 percent agreed that their desire to study basic science was increased by the preceptorship.

At the end of the preceptorships, students have consistently exhibited great enthusiasm for returning to the medical school to pursue their basic science learning. The original curricular design called for IB to begin after nine months of the first year of medical school. The first two classes, upon returning from their preceptorship, felt that it was so important in helping them understand the need for basic sciences, and for placing their learning in perspective, that they requested it commence after the first six and one-half months of school. PCC planners granted the request. This has allowed two additional months for basic science tutorials to be moved into the second year prior to the students taking the National Board examination. Despite a shortened Phase IA preparation, the first class to go through this new schedule had one of the better experiences in IB.

The stresses of being at remote sites during Phase IB were not fully anticipated by faculty or students. Starting a new job, moving to a new community, and making new friends is stressful for anyone. It is particularly true in a highly pressured field like medicine. The following comments were given in response to a question asking for the negative aspects of IB:

> *"Three problems: Distance of the Questa Health Center where I worked from the hospital activities, trying to find enough time to work on a community project, and not having anyone to discuss basic sciences with."*

> *"It was hard not having another student to bounce ideas, concerns, and frustrations off of while at the preceptorship site."*

> *"At times I spent too much time in the clinic (my fault). Yet there was no special room set aside for me to study in the clinic. I felt too pressured to complete my community project."*

The 16-week duration of the Phase IB preceptorship creates a special strain on some of the married students. Though spouses are encouraged to move to the preceptorship sites, many are working and unable to leave their jobs. The program has responded to this problem by offering counseling to the couples and by facilitating peer discussions of these problems among the students.

Where possible, the program is flexible in accommodating the students' noneducational needs. Almost 10 percent of the students have been offered preceptorships in the Albuquerque area in order to help meet their legitimate personal needs. Even though the sites of these preceptorships are more urban-based than the program prefers, the importance of accommodating individual needs provides the kind of program sensitivity it hopes the students will incorporate into their own attitudes as future practitioners.

One unanticipated result of Phase IB has been its capacity to identify problem students. Although there were questions about these students during their pre-IB experience, the tutorial environment was able to support the student through the units. It was not until the preceptorship, when students were more on their own, that their problems became clearly manifested. In each of these cases individualized interventions were necessary, including removing the student from the preceptorship site and tailoring study plans to meet particular student deficiencies. In each case the problems have been of the type that may have escaped notice in traditional, lecture-based, basic science courses, only to surface during the clinical years. But because of the individual attention to students that characterizes PCC, earlier intervention for students in difficulty has been possible.

Earlier classes of PCC students have given important feedback to the program about the importance of the rural preceptorship to later medical school experiences. Not only has it enhanced their subsequent basic science learning, but it has provided an important point of reference during their later hospital clerkship rotations. When attendings would badger students on rounds, or colleagues would confide their dismay at doing mindless "scut work," PCC students could reflect on IB and say, "I know it isn't really like this out in practice." They felt better anchored by their prior, "real world" experience.

Effects of Rural Preceptorship on PCC. Student experience with the first few years of Phase IB has resulted in two major alterations. The first, discussed above, was the earlier timing of the Phase IB within the curriculum. The second is the pairing of students in community sites. The faculty who set up the first preceptor–student matches paid too little attention to the students' need for peer support. Students were, for the most part, placed individually in preceptorship locations which were geographically removed from one another. However, too many students felt socially and educationally isolated. Therefore, beginning with the third class, students were paired in a community (or assigned as a group in one geographic area) so that they could meet with one another on a regular basis.

A surprising aspect of the IB program was the high motivation with which students pursued cultural, social, and psychological issues in the field. These areas had been relatively neglected on campus. Engel (1977) has long admonished medical educators to broaden their teaching framework to incorporate a biopsychosocial model of illness. Yet PCC has found that when tutorial groups work on case problems at the medical school, even on those problems specifically designed to pique the students' interest in psychosocial issues, discussion drifts magnetically toward conventional basic science topics. Whether it is because of the ubiquitousness of the campus-based basic science faculty, the proximate basic science lectures for traditional-track students, or the gnawing perception of the upcoming National Board examination, students clearly seem distracted from the broader social issues inherent in their case problems.

The students' blossoming interest in broader issues when living in communities is expressed not only by the learning issues generated from their patient contacts, but the breadth of thought exhibited in their community research projects. One student, for example, was working in a Hispanic community in northern New Mexico which suffered from high unemployment. A cottage industry of boarding homes had sprung up around the nearby State Mental Hospital to care for ex-patients, 80 percent of whom never returned to their home community. The student was intrigued and made the following observation:

> *"A person seen wandering aimlessly around town giving off an aura of having nowhere in particular to be, and nothing in particular to do, more than likely lives in one of the many boarding homes located around the city. This person is probably on Social Security or Supplemental Security Income. This person pays most of his income to the boarding-home owner, who is in charge of his shelter, food, clothing, and general welfare."*

The student conducted a survey of 100 ex-patients, many boarding-home operators, and a sampling of the general public to determine their attitudes toward the plight of the chronically mentally ill in their midst. He found that in ex-patients' home communities there was a paucity of local mental health resources, and frequently a problem of family burn-out. However, in this community there was a very strong network of local community support for these people. The student developed this theme with sensitivity and insight. The work is characteristic of the genuine interest in the social dimensions of community health problems that are exhibited by PCC students in their sustained rural clerkships.

What We Have Learned

1. Longitudinal community preceptorships, in either urban or rural communities, can be an important component of medical students' education during their preclinical years.
2. To maximize the importance of the educational experience, students should offer useful clinical service under supervision, while they learn.
3. Students should be prepared with skills in such subjects as biostatistics, epidemiology, and health economics to appreciate fully the social forces affecting an individual's health

and to be capable of conducting a community health assessment.

4. Sites should be selected in which the preceptor displays the qualities eventually expected of the students (e.g., working well with the health care team, treating patients holistically, being involved in preventive services for the community, and being a lifelong learner).

5. A plan of educational resource support for the community-based students should be developed, including special library access, circuit riders, and telephone consultation backup.

6. A comprehensive student evaluation mechanism should be instituted during the preceptorship, because its length provides a unique setting in which to observe closely student strengths and weaknesses and to remedy the latter.

Experience at Other Schools

Since 1971, the University of Minnesota Medical School has offered third-year students the option of an extended, rural preceptorship lasting nine to 12 months. It offers perhaps the most extensive problem-based field experience to students and has had the longest track record in this area of any medical school. Students work in rural primary-care settings and in rural hospitals. Students and their families live in their rural communities while in the program. Preceptors include either family physicians or internists (Garrard & Verby, 1977). The goal of this Rural Physician Associate Program (RPAP) is to provide an intensive, long-term experience in rural health care for third-year students, encouraging the eventual practice of medicine in a rural setting. This innovation was an outgrowth of a curricular revision instituted in 1969, in which students in the third and fourth year selected one of seven specialty tracks, each featuring a unique cluster of courses.

To compare the experience of RPAP students to those taking conventional third-year hospital ward clerkships, students in each group completed a detailed, coded, patient-encounter form for a seven-month period. Statistical differences between the two groups were found on almost all variables studied. RPAP students saw triple the number of patients, performed double the number of clinical procedures, and were given far greater responsibility. The groups also saw a different mix of patients. For example, the five leading conditions seen by RPAP students in rural clinics were fractures, lacerations, congestive heart failure, hypertension, and pregnancy. In contrast, the most common illnesses seen by University hospital-based students were alcoholism, cerebrovascular accident, angina pectoris, congestive heart failure, and psychosis.

Program directors concluded that a long-term preceptorship in a primary-care setting provides students with a patient population more representative of the community and offers a richer clinical experience (Verby et al., 1981). Students in the field do not have to compete with each other for clinical experience, a problem which bedevils clinical education in the trainee-glutted tertiary-care university hospitals. Another advantage of the long-term preceptorship is the students' greater ability to follow patients over time. Long-term follow-up facilitates a stronger student–patient relationship, and the student is motivated to study the patient's clinical problem in much greater depth.

As in PCC, the Minnesota group finds the extended rural preceptorship to be advantageous for student evaluation.

> It allows the teacher/student relationship to extend for such a length that the student's cognitive and stylistic strengths and weaknesses can be identified. In a short-term rotation, it is often difficult to gain an accurate perception of the student's deficiencies. (Verby et al., 1981, p. 646)

The RPAP student receives a $10,000 stipend for his year of rural education (half paid by the State, half by the physician preceptor). As in the New Mexico program, University of Minnesota faculty visit the sites on a monthly basis but serve a consulting role for the community physicians as well as the student. The program has thus built bridges of goodwill between the University and the rural communities (Heid, 1979).

Implications

An extended community-based preceptorship during the early years of medical school can enhance the goals of a problem-based curriculum. The principles of problem-based learning that were gained in tutorial groups with simulated problems on campus can now be applied to a sustained, real-life setting in which the student must function more independently.

Sustained community-based experiences can begin in "preclinical" years or early in the clinical years. They can be organized as several individual time blocks or as long-term, student–community affiliations. In each case the experience presents students with a far broader exposure to the health care delivery system, and to the multiple forces affecting illness in the community.

By placing students in a more independent, responsible role in the community, important individual strengths can be developed and built on, and weaknesses can be uncovered and dealt with constructively. These student qualities would usually be masked in a conventional lecture-based curriculum, or even in an on-campus, small-group tutorial program.

References

Engel, G. L. (1977, April 8). A need for a new medical model: A challenge for biomedicine. *Science, 196,* 129–136.

Garrard, J., & Verby, J. E. (1977). Comparison of medical student experiences in rural and university settings. *Journal of Medical Education, 52,* 802–810.

Harris, D. L., & Elbert, P. J. (1983). Effects of clinical preceptorship on career and practice site choices. *Western Journal of Medicine, 138* (2), 276–79.

Heid, J. K. (1979). Rural Physician Associate Program—a boon to rural Minnesota. *Minnesota Medicine, 62,* 826–828.

Mullan F. (1982). Community-oriented primary care: An agenda for the '80s. *New England Journal of Medicine, 307,* 1076–1078.

Paiva, R. E. A. (1982). Effect of clinical experiences in medical school on specialty choice decisions. *Journal of Medical Education, 57,* 666–674.

Quenk N., & Smith S. (1976). *From initiation to evaluation: Developing primary care preceptorships.* Albuquerque: American Medical Student Association Foundation.

Verby J. E., Schaefer, M. T., & Voeks R. S. (1981). Learning forestry out of the lumberyard. *Journal of the American Medical Association, 246,* 645–647.

CHAPTER 8

Evaluating Student Performance

DONALD A. WEST, BERTHOLD E. UMLAND, AND SUSAN M. LUCERO

"Those who control the examinations control the entire curriculum." The anonymous author of this observation wisely understood that the real goals of an educational program are determined by, and discernible from, the evaluation system. Put another way: what is measured is what is, or becomes, valued. (Jason & Westberg, 1982, p. 101)

Goals of Student Evaluation in a Problem-Based Curriculum

1. *Evaluation geared to program goals.* Evaluation methods should be broad enough to provide feedback to the program and to its students on the degree to which program goals are being achieved by students.
2. *Congruence between methods of evaluation and medical practice.* To optimize the value of evaluation to the student's future career, its methods should adequately assess those skills the student is expected to demonstrate in later practice.

3. *Evaluation of process more than content.* Evaluation should emphasize assessment of problem solving and application of knowledge, rather than assessment of accumulated facts.
4. *Provision of informal as well as formal evaluation.* A student's evaluation should be both informal (frequent, less formal feedback enabling continuous remediation) and formal (end of course, more formal, often "after the fact") to afford the student maximum feedback and opportunity for improvement.

Introduction

Medical education is plagued by an almost exclusive reliance on fact-oriented, multiple-choice, and short-answer examinations to evaluate students in their preclinical years. The need for different methods of instruction and evaluation that focus more on problem solving and knowledge application has been well documented (Bishop, 1984; Bloom, 1956; Erdmann, 1982; Jason, 1974; Obenshain, 1982). But this need has been overshadowed by two powerful forces: a pervasive thirst on the part of faculty for quantification and the influence on medical schools of the National Board of Medical Examiners.

"How can we know what they're learning if we can't measure it?" This is the reasoning of many educators for whom the National Board provides the reassurance of a national standard, no matter that it is unrelated to the unique goals of any particular institution. In violation of the stated intent of the National Board, medical schools are increasingly using the examination for internal promotion of students rather than as an external evaluation of one component of department effectiveness in teaching.

Evaluators instead should ask several crucial questions: What abilities and skills should a graduating medical student have? How can they be assessed? How well does the present evaluation system assess them? A proposal developed by the National Board of Medical Examiners for their Comprehensive Qualifying exam for licensure (AAMC Ad Hoc External Examination Review Committee, 1981) identified ten "tasks" and five "abilities" which the board believed should be performed competently by any physician entering graduate medical education (Figure 8.1). With their specially developed techniques including latent image clinical problem techniques, the NBME stated that it could assess 12 of the 50 cells in the matrix. If one ponders the matrix more soberly to see how many cells are routinely assessed by widely accepted

Figure 8.1.   Modified matrix of tasks and abilities deemed necessary for physicians entering graduate medical education.*

ABILITIES TASKS	A Knowledge and Understanding	B Problem–Solving and Judgement	C Technical Skills	D Interpersonal skills	E Work Habits and Attitude
1. Taking a history	MCQ**				
2. Performing a physical examination	MCQ				
3. Using diagnostic aids	MCQ				
4. Defining problems	MCQ				
5. Managing therapy	MCQ				
6. Keeping records					
7. Employing special sources of information					
8. Monitoring and maintaining health	MCQ				
9. Assuming community and professional responsibilities					
10. Maintaining professional competence					

*From AAMC Hoc External Examinaution Review Commitee (1981). A critical analysis and alternative method, part II, External Examination for the evaluation of medical education achievement and for licensure. Journal of Medical Education, 56, 947.

**MCQ refers to multiple choice question examinations.

fact-recall examinations, a generous estimate would be only 5 of the 50 cells.

In his extensive review of the validity of multiple-choice-question (MCQ) examinations, the kind most widely used in medical schools, Neufeld (1984) concludes: "There are no convincing studies that demonstrate the predictive validity of MCQ examinations."

To make matters worse, grades derived from MCQ examinations bear little or no correlation with later performance as a physician (Wingard & Williamson, 1973). Since traditional evaluation methods have severe limitations when assessing what is needed to be a physician, it is important to scrutinize how problem-based learning programs have attempted to select and develop evaluation instruments to assess their students' achievement of program goals.

University of New Mexico Program

Background

Although the PCC evaluation scheme was initially based on instruments developed at McMaster University in Canada, circumstances unique to the University of New Mexico required considerable modification of these instruments over time. PCC contended with the existence of a well-established, traditional, lecture-based curriculum in the first two years, a factor which McMaster did not have to consider. UNM's dual track generated inevitable comparisons. Faculty skepticism as to the practicality of the PCC approach required an evaluation system that was both appropriate to the problem-based, tutorial method and credible to a faculty familiar with, and oriented toward, written, memory-based, multiple-choice, fact-oriented exams.

Since the philosophical underpinnings of PCC gave preeminence to the processes of learning, reasoning, and information seeking, evaluation focused on these elements more than on measuring factual knowledge.

Tutorial Evaluation

Tutorial groups were strongly encouraged to reserve time at the end of each meeting to informally evaluate the contribution of each member (including the tutor).

Formal evaluation took place at the midpoint and end of each eight-week tutorial unit. Forms were designed for students to evaluate their own performances in the areas of knowledge base, clinical reasoning, evaluation skills, and fulfillment of a personal learning plan. Each student was expected to rate all of the members of the group, including the tutor, and to share this material openly at the mid- and end-unit meetings. Such meetings were usually held at a group member's home in the evening, after a potluck dinner, and might last up to six hours. Faculty tutors were expected subsequently to read over the comments and ratings and corroborate or make minor additions to each student's self-evaluation.

The evaluation meetings were often emotionally charged affairs as students and tutors gave honest feedback about interpersonal as well as academic performance. Depending on the group's history, feedback could be given with "kid gloves" or could be brutally frank. Significant positive change in individual and group performance was usually evident after the mid-unit evaluation session.

It gradually became apparent that evaluation of an individual student solely in such group sessions was inadequate. The talkative, assertive, and personable students could push their strengths and often mask their weakness. The shy or quiet students sometimes appeared not to have mastered material discussed by other students. At times, if the group dynamics were not comfortable for some students they might "tune out" or fail to encourage a slower student.

Concern over the Students' Knowledge Base. During the first few years, students with less faith in the problem-based method expressed concern about the adequacy of their knowledge. They questioned whether the method was allowing them to learn and retain what they needed since they had none of the familiar benchmarks of the conventional curriculum: examination scores. A student in the first class recounted the following conversation between two students: "Are we learning anything?" "Let's not worry! We *must* be learning something, the PCC faculty know what they're doing." The faculty often felt that they, themselves, were "flying by the seat of their pants" and counting on the students' intelligence and enthusiasm to bring about favorable results.

The tutors also expressed a concern that if they felt that a particular student was not doing well, there was no mechanism to confirm or deny that impression.

External Skepticism. While PCC students and faculty basked in the program's novelty, non-PCC faculty began to express concern about the students. Many felt that a tutor could not be expected to evaluate a student's knowledge adequately in a basic science discipline remote from that tutor's expertise. How could an anatomist, for example, adequately evaluate a student's command of biochemistry? An attitude developed on the part of some faculty skeptics that PCC was trying to "put one over on us" by letting students get by without rigorous testing and by keeping unfavorable data from the conventional faculty. To address the uneasiness of both faculty and students, PCC planners developed evaluation tools that were more objective.

Objective Examinations

Students in each track at UNM are required to take and pass the NBME Part I examination at the end of the second year before promotion to the third year, regardless of prior academic performance. While conventional-track students repeatedly received tests similar in format to

NBME throughout the courses in their first two years, PCC students had no comparable preparation.

Thus, during the second year of the PCC program, a decision to provide quantitative feedback was made. The Quarterly Profile Exam (QPE) (Willoughby & Hutcheson, 1978) was purchased from the University of Missouri–Kansas City (UMKC) and offered to all of the PCC students on a quarterly basis.* The examination seemed to be an ideal tool for PCC because its test items were selected from all basic science areas as well as major clinical areas. It was also designed to be comprehensive so students could not "cram" for it and could be credited for *any* area in medicine they may have chosen to study. It had also been field-tested extensively at UMKC, permitting statistical analysis of scores between students in PCC and students at a comparable level at UMKC. The examination showed promise of predicting which students were at risk for failing Part I of NBME, and it could thus be used to identify students who required special remedial assistance.

There were some immediate problems with the QPE. The examination was not initially required, so not all of the students took it. Although the examination was short enough that it took only one day to administer, its brevity became a disadvantage because each constituent part of the scoring analysis was based on only a few items (e.g., the biochemistry score might reflect answers to only 10 or 15 questions). Further, the basic science faculty who analyzed the examination felt that too many of the questions were poorly written or not important. Whether this represented institutional pride, condescension, or careful analysis was debatable.

During the two years that the students took the QPE, there was a good correlation between the QPE and the subsequent passage of Part I of the National Boards. Lack of an upward trend in scores on the QPE was thus used to identify students with problems in comprehension, retention, or test-taking ability. PCC could intervene early, before a student failed the Boards.

Eventually, however, the students and faculty expressed enough dissatisfaction with the QPE that PCC made a decision to substitute the Shelf Boards.† The Shelf Boards are old National Board examinations that are sold by the NBME at the price of $15 per subject per student. If 20 or more students take the exam at one time, a full statistical analysis

---

*The test can be purchased from: Cashier's Office, University of Missouri, 5100 Rockhill Rd., Kansas City, MO 64110.
†Shelf Boards can be purchased from the National Board of Medical Examiners, 3930 Chestnut, Philadelphia, PA 19104.

of each group's performance in relation to those who have taken that test nationally is made available to the program. Selection of the Shelf Boards was a judicious decision both politically and practically. The correlation of the Shelf Boards with passage of the National Board of Medical Examiners—Part I is high, and among the students and faculty there was credibility, for it was already recognized as the "gold standard."

Currently, all PCC students in the first two years are required to take the Shelf Boards every six months. Thus, each student will have taken them a minimum of three times by the end of the second year, when all students must take the National Boards for promotion. A student who does not feel confident about taking the National Boards can take the Shelf Boards a fourth time in the summer, and then take the Boards for credit in the fall.

No PCC class has thus far taken the Shelf Boards on all four administrations, yet three classes have taken parts of the Shelf Board Series (Figure 8.2). Data from these tests show a trend in expected scores which will be useful in counseling students in their first year about how well they are doing in comparison to previous students in preparation for this examination. It is especially useful for students who score poorly on their last Shelf Examination in January of their second year and are considered "high risk." They can see expected trends in scores from students who have fared comparably in prior years and plan special remediation for delay of the National Board examination until the end of the summer (Figure 8.3).

Individual Process Assessment

The IPA is a comprehensive exercise designed to give each student an opportunity to be evaluated on the full range of activities expected of a physician. The student must assess a clinical problem using a simulated patient; utilize history-taking and physical examination skills; identify a patient's problems and develop hypotheses about the mechanisms that might be causing the problems; test the hypotheses by ordering laboratory and radiologic examinations and other ancillary tests; revise the hypotheses by incorporating the new information in the patient's data base; then discuss with a clinical and basic scientist evaluator team the approach to the problems, how the conclusions were reached, and what new information was learned during the study. The IPA takes a little over 50 hours (Figure 8.4).

The faculty is expected to observe with the student at least part of the 50-minute videotaped encounter between the student and simulated

Figure 8.2. Scores on NBME Shelf examination and NBME—Part I for three classes of PCC students.

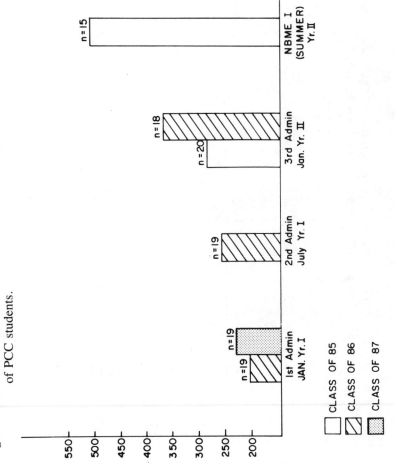

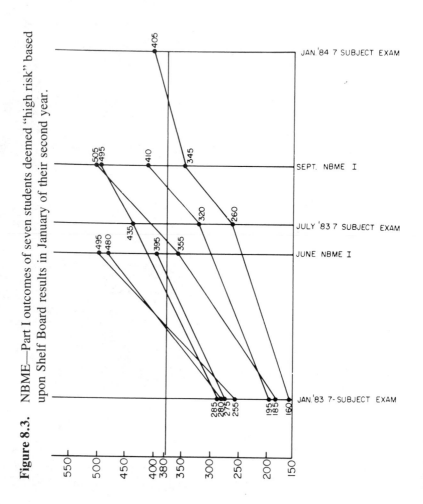

Figure 8.3. NBME—Part I outcomes of seven students deemed "high risk" based upon Shelf Board results in January of their second year.

Figure 8.4. Outline of Individual Process Assessment (IPA).

50 MINUTES

> Student interviews and examines simulated patient.

> Student lists and ranks identified problems; ranks and supports hypotheses.

> Student obtains investigative results and costs (Room B65A).*

*You must obtain your results in 3 hours. Please bring lab result printout to your review session.

> Student writes as complete data base on patient as possible.

48 HOURS

> Student lists areas of knowledge, strengths, and learning issues.

> Student studies case, making any desired changes on above documentation.*

*Use different color of pen/pencil

> Student turns in documentation to PCC office 1½ hours prior to evaluation or at 8 A.M.

1 HOUR & 45 MINUTES

> Student presents/discusses case with evaluator(s).

> Evaluator(s)/student cosign narrative assessment of performance; student evaluates IPA.*

*This documentation should be turned in to B-80 within 24 hours after review.

24 HOURS

> Further discussion & exploration of case occurs in tutorial group with "model" documentation available to the group.

patient and to critique the student's bedside manner, interviewing style, and physical examination technique. Other staff members observe the entire interaction during the videotaping and fill out a checklist about what information was obtained, what interpersonal skills were evidenced, and how thoroughly the physical examination was performed. In addition, the simulated patient fills out an evaluation of the student. This feedback is first given to the student verbally at the end of the encounter, and later in writing when the student meets with the faculty evaluators.

For the purposes of this examination, a correct diagnosis is less important than the student's ability to think through the data in a systematic manner and to be able to explain the mechanisms by which hypothesized causes could explain the presenting complaints. While the students are often anxious about the IPAs and devote heroic efforts to them in a compressed time frame, afterwards they usually say they have learned a great deal, not only about the particular issues that they studied, but also about the process of reasoning.

The IPA duplicates a real-world clinical experience so faithfully that PCC students on third-year clinical rotations look back on IPAs as one of their best preparations for clinical medicine. One student summarized the feelings of many:

> *"You know those IPAs were a bear and I dreaded them every time. But in retrospect they really prepared me for the wards. Every day is just like having another IPA—you do a huge amount of work in a very short time. It's probably logistically impossible, but it would be ideal if PCC students in the first and second year could do one every week or two."*

Although initially committed to the administration of an IPA at the end of every tutorial unit, and to the evaluation of each student by an experienced clinician and a basic scientist, program administrators found that resources would not stretch that far. Despite the IPAs potential for evaluation of the students' mastery of virtually every program objective, it is enormously labor intensive. To conduct IPAs for 20 students in one week requires approximately 200 hours of staff time and at least 80 hours of faculty time—all in the space of a few days.

There has also been some difficulty ascribing a precise level of performance to a student on such a complex evaluation. At the outset, the scale on which all students were graded ranged from: "unsatisfactory for first-year student" to "outstanding for graduating senior student." While program planners were proud of their unique evaluation design, the first-year student who was given a passing grade called "unsatisfactory for a second-year student" felt crushed. With this ambiguity, interrater reliability was nil. As a consequence, a simplified scoring scale with room for narrative evaluation is now used. Five categories are assessed: Clinical Skills, Recording/Presenting, Reasoning, Knowledge Base, and Behavioral Skills. Students are rated in each category on a scale from 0 to 4 ("Unsatisfactory" to "Outstanding"). Eventually, the program administrators hope to develop a criterion-based reference system combined with some faculty-defined minimums of acceptable performance.

There are two lingering problems with the IPA. There remains enormous discomfort on the part of many basic scientists when paired with clinicians to evaluate students in areas with which the basic scientists have little experience. While many basic scientists are eager to learn and participate, some withdraw into near-silence during the evaluation, and some request not to participate again. The program's intensive efforts to orient the basic scientists to the issues in each case before the actual evaluation have ameliorated the problem somewhat. But careful selection of basic scientists with more positive attitudes toward this experiment has been even more helpful.

Finally, interrater reliability remains variable, as is evaluator adherence to a standard format expected by the students. Despite careful preparation, some evaluators cannot resist badgering students on their content knowledge to the exclusion of other aspects of their evaluation, while others are comfortable only discussing areas within their own expertise. The evaluation planners feel a tension between competing goals. PCC is interested in faculty development—to give faculty an opportunity to improve their evaluation skills; yet the goals of students' learning call for contact with "only the best" evaluators. This issue is not yet resolved.

Need for Order: An Evaluation Committee Is Formed

During the first year of the program, faculty and staff were so excited and awed by their first class that the students were treated as precious objects whose every activity was dutifully noted and transcribed. But no one was certain what should be done with the accumulating data. Each student's file, in the Office of Student Affairs, became thicker . . . and thicker.

While PCC planners were proud of this full documentation and evaluation of each student's progress, the Dean of Student Affairs found that wading through the unsummarized file material was a chaotic, tedious experience of little value. In the small group setting tutors often became personally attached to their students. As a consequence many lost objectivity and had difficulty giving an unsatisfactory grade. It was so much easier to be an objective grader when your student had not become a friend and colleague.

The problem was compounded by a lack of firm evaluation criteria for the categories being evaluated. Further, because of PCC's philosophy of fostering cooperation rather than competition, the "superior" grades given in the conventional track were initially not given in PCC, further blurring distinction between students. Tutors' skills at evaluating in this relatively new tutorial setting were so variable that students lacked consistent feedback on their performance.

Finally, many students were reluctant to assume responsibility for recommending a failing grade to a fellow student. They felt that was an unfair burden on them which should be the program's responsibility.

One senior PCC student reflected,

> *"Sometimes tutors didn't give students clear messages. It's a disservice when they 'support' students too much over initial bumps that should be felt much harder. And I think tutors have got to find a way of being both supportive and hard-ass. It's difficult to do because you develop a relationship in those tutorials and that relationship is strongly reinforced around being colleagues, friendly, and so forth. It takes a lot of skill to find that balance, to do both."*

Thus an Evaluation Committee, formed early in the fourth year of the program, was charged with making the process of evaluation more forthright, coherent, and better organized. The members of this committee, selected for their reputations for order and decisiveness, talked to the students individually about their progress and arranged remedial programs if necessary. While tutors now submit recommended grades on the basis of the tutorial group's evaluation, it is the Evaluation Committee that assigns the final grade, thereby applying greater objectivity.

Remedial Intervention

Considerable faculty time was expended in developing methods to intervene in an appropriate and timely manner when students encounter difficulties. The traditional method of giving a repeat written examination with an arbitrary pass–fail level was neither appropriate nor possible since the PCC students in difficulty were not failing objective written tests. Instead, they were having problems in group interaction or were not developing skills in problem solving or identification of learning issues.

As the program evolved, more creative, individualized, and usually successful methods were developed to allow earlier intervention. For example, students who had poor scores on the QPE were sometimes required to take and pass upper-division, undergraduate basic science courses before being promoted. Psychiatric counseling was recommended when it was evident that personal turmoil was having an adverse effect on academic or interpersonal performance in tutorial groups. Students who exhibited difficulty reasoning "on their feet" in tutorials were asked to meet weekly before tutorial sessions, with faculty members. The faculty would rehearse the students at these meetings by firing questions at them, helping them to become accustomed to reasoning impromptu. For students with unsatisfactory performance on IPAs, focused remediation in the clinical problem-solving areas was devised. These students were assigned to a supervising clinician who would arrange one patient encounter per week, allowing the student to practice clinical skills, clinical reasoning, and case presentation. This individualized tutoring went on simultaneously with the group tutorials and other curriculum activities.

As one reviewed the PCC students who had had difficulties, one could see a pattern gradually emerging. They were predominantly individuals who could not look clearly at themselves, assess their problems, or take responsibility for themselves and their own learning. They were students with strong defenses against low self-esteem who made great use of denial. They often tended to be "loners" with tenuous ties to other tutorial group members. While many of their problems would have gone unnoticed in the anonymity of a lecture hall, the close scrutiny of peers and faculty in a tutorial group or rural clerkship resulted in their difficulties being identified early.

What We Have Learned

1. *It is critical to identify program goals before selecting evaluation instruments.* First determine which skills and knowledge students should ideally exhibit upon graduation. Then select or develop evaluation instruments to assess the students' proficiency in those areas.
2. *There is considerable time saved by sampling evaluation forms and instruments from other problem-based pro-*

grams. It is far easier and much less costly to utilize or modify evaluation materials already developed by other problem-based programs than to create such materials de novo.

3. *It is important to select diverse evaluation methods.* The use of multiple evaluation methods provides a fuller and more accurate assessment of each student and better identifies areas needing remediation.

4. *To ensure objectivity, it is important to establish an independent evaluation committee.* A separate committee should be established to design and implement evaluation methods and review all components of a student's evaluation. This will provide the objectivity needed to balance the tendency toward subjectivity engendered by a problem-based tutorial program.

5. *It is important to include content as well as process evaluations.* There is a tendency, in a problem-based program, to emphasize the student's reasoning and problem-solving abilities and interpersonal skills to the exclusion of his or her knowledge of content. This is a serious mistake. Such exclusive emphasis fails to adequately assess the degree to which the curriculum is conveying factual information and the ability of the students to learn it.

6. *The student-centered philosophy of learning is reinforced by letting student share responsibility for their evaluation.* Students must share responsibility for self and peer evaluation in oral and written form if lifelong skills in this domain are to be developed. Althcugh students should not have sole responsibility, the program should ensure that their input is more than cursory.

Experience at Other Schools

Evaluation for McMaster University medical students is viewed as an integral part of the learning system rather than as a separate set of events (Neufeld, 1982). Tutorial assessment occurs informally as self, peer, and tutor assessment. In the preclinical years, it occurs primarily during tutorial by use of an instrument called the Triple Jump (Powles, et al., 1981). The Triple Jump is an assessment in three steps: problem definition, information search, and synthesis. The evaluation is conducted by nontutor faculty.

Evaluations are also obtained from clinical skills preceptors. The tutor for the unit collects all the evaluations and prepares a summary of each student's performance in the areas of knowledge and problem-solving, professional characteristices, and self-directed learning ability. The statement and documentation are reviewed by the unit planner. There are no traditional grades or ranking. However, if a student accumulates two "unsatisfactories," a faculty review board conducts a review of the student's record and determines an appropriate course of action.

After 13 years of experience, the strengths of the McMaster program evaluation system seem to be the consistency between what is taught and what is assessed. Feedback to students is continual, evaluation methods are varied, and learning is stressed during evaluation.

Drawbacks of the assessment program are, in some ways, a result of the very same consistency between curriculum and evaluation. Students and faculty in the program cite problems resulting from the tendency toward subjectivity in the evaluations. Students have difficulty balancing the need for factual recall with their own "process" objectives.

The Michigan State University (MSU) evaluation scheme for students in their problem-based "Track 2" is of three types:

1.   A narrative evaluation completed by small-group faculty preceptors at the end of each term. This is similar to New Mexico's tutor evaluation.
2.   A problem-solving evaluation given twice each term, in which students work through clinical cases sequentially, responding to various types of problem-solving questions with written narrative responses. This is usually done as an open-book, take-home exercise and graded by small-group faculty preceptors against preset criteria for each response.
3.   Content examinations consisting of multiple-choice and matching questions which include items from all disciplines (Jones et al., 1983).

Performance is monitored by the Track 2 director, with periodic formal review by the 27-person Track 2 Committee using all available evaluation components. The committee makes recommendations for modification of any student's program, if necessary.

Program evaluators for Track 2 compare the program to McMaster (see above) and cite the use of the content examination as the major difference between the two programs. The difference arose as a result of a threat by conventional, Track 1 faculty, that they would support Track 2 only if the content studied and evaluated was essentially the same as that of Track 1.

The MSU group feels that the importance of the content examination for each of their focal problems has been overemphasized. The structure is often more apparent than real. Where some students use the tests as the central focus of study, as in most traditional curricula, the flexibility in the timing of examinations allows others a leeway in determining when they have mastered the content, allowing for some degree of student self-assessment in a faculty-imposed evaluation system. Jones et al. find important advantages for their open-book, take-home problem assessment evaluation given twice a term:

> A significant advantage of the open-book, take-home method of administration is that it is possible to assess the student's ability to use resources as aids in problem-solving, rather than assessing only the student's recall. Also, there are fewer constraints on realism than are present with the in-class administered case or for the classic patient management problem. It is possible to provide much more extensive patient data, to follow the patient over an extended period of time, and to include clinical problems that have not as yet been studied. (Jones et al., 1983, p. 22)

The method of assessment of problem-based learning at the University of Newcastle Medical School in Australia has been extensively reported in the literature. This assessment is performed using an instrument known as the Modified Essay Question (MEQ) (Feletti & Engel, 1980; Hodgkin & Knox, 1975), a serial, structured, question examination presenting a clinical case in sequence. Each page adds new clinical information and asks a question requiring an essay-type response and a decision. To simulate the actual clinical situation, previewing items in the booklet (looking forward) or turning back to change answers once new data are presented are both prohibited. The sequence includes items requiring interpretation of X-rays, microscopic sections, and videotaped segments of a patient's behavior.

Following administration of the MEQ at the end of each term, time is allotted for evaluators to have extensive oral interviews with students whose papers contain "doubtful" answers. Students deemed not satisfactory at the end of the interview are given two additional attempts with a pair of evaluators during the remainder of the year when the student feels prepared. These later assessments cover the student's identified areas of weakness. A final deferred assessment is compulsory for all students still not judged satisfactory by the end of the academic year. Only then is a "pass" or "fail" recorded. Students with two or more "fails" in the same year would normally be expelled or would begin in a special study program.

The MEQ has been found to be reliable and valid (Feletti, 1980b). Newcastle faculty believe it has proven invaluable for diagnosing student weaknesses and for providing a concrete basis for remediation. It has the advantage of being criterion referenced. And since it is standardized, it obviates the many problems with interrater reliability found in New Mexico's IPA while still examining problem-solving skills.

Southern Illinois University uses three innovative evaluation tools:

1. The Clinical Reasoning Test is a written exam using problem-based learning modules and administered three times during the year. This method has the advantages of testing the reasoning process and requiring little faculty time to score (Williams et al., 1983).

2. With the multiple-station exercise, all students circulate to various stations at each of which a specific, problem-solving task is required of them (Chapter 5). They may be asked to interpret an X-ray of a patient with pneumonia or to interview a simulated epileptic patient who is requesting medical evaluation to obtain a driver's license. This has been extremely successful in providing an assessment of integration of knowledge and skills.

3. Practical instructors are actual or simulated patients trained to be examined by students, to discuss the aspects of their actual or simulated disorders, to evaluate the examination, and to teach ways to improve the examination. They are used at SIU to assess clinical skills not only in Sequence II but in the clinical year as well. Practical instructors have the advantage of making the assessment a learning experience and have the potential to reduce the demand on faculty time and therefore the cost of medical education. The initial cost of training them, however, is substantial, as it is with any simulated patients.

Implications

Designing and implementing evaluation methods which are consistent with a problem-based approach and which evaluate problem solving has been a challenge. But all of the schools discussed have developed instruments which are being used and are providing valuable data about student performance and abilities. A number of these, particularly the pencil-and-paper tools (e.g., the Modified Essay Question and the Clinical Reasoning Test), are easily scored and criterion referenced. Evaluation in tutorial groups and by direct observation is less reliable and more variable (in general), but provides valuable data not otherwise available, such as a student's interpersonal skills. The varieties of evaluation being developed and successfully utilized belie the view that the traditional multiple-choice/objective examination is the best way of evaluating preclinical students.

References

AAMC Ad Hoc External Examination Review Committee. (1981). A critical analysis and alternative method. Part II of External examination for the evaluation of medical education achievement and for licensure. *Journal of Medical Education, 56,* 957.

Bishop, J. M. (1984). Infuriating tensions: Science and the medical student. *Journal of Medical Education, 59,* 91–102.

Bloom, B. S. (1956). *Taxonomy of educational objectives: The classification of goals, Handbook I (Cognitive Domains).* London, Longmans Green.

Erdmann, J. B. (1982). Testing evaluation and teaching the new biology. In C. P. Freidman & E. F. Purcell (Eds.), *The new biology in medical education: Merging the biological information and cognitive sciences* (pp. 236–242). New York: Josiah Macy, Jr. Foundation.

Feletti, G. I. (1980a). Evaluation of a comprehensive programme for the assessment of medical students. *Higher Education, 9,* 169–178.

Feletti, G. I. (1980b). Reliability and validity studies on modified essay questions. *Journal of Medical Education, 55,* 933–941.

Feletti, G. I., & Engel, C. E. (1980). The modified essay question for testing problem-solving skills. *Medical Journal of Australia, 1,* 79–80.

Hodgkin, K., & Knox, J. D. (1975). *Problem-centered learning.* London: Churchill Livingstone.

Jason, H. (1974). Evaluation of basic science learning: Implications of and for the GAP Report. Editorial. *Journal of Medical Education, 49,* 1003–1004.

Jason, H., & Westberg, J. (1982). *Teachers and Teaching in U.S. Medical Schools.* Norwalk, Conn.: Appleton-Century-Crofts.

Jones, J. W., Bieber, L. L., Echt, R., Schiefley, V., & Ways, P. O. (1983). A problem-based curriculum—Ten years of experience. Maastricht Annual Research in Problem-Based Learning Conference.

Neufeld, V. R. (1982) Student assessment in medical education: A Canadian case study. *Assessment and Evaluation in Higher Education, 7,* 203–215.

Neufeld, V. R. (1984). Written examinations in clinical competence. In V. R. Neufeld & G. R. Norman (Eds.), *Assessing clinical competence.* New York: Springer Publishing Company.

Obenshain, S. S. (1982). Old wine in new skins: Teaching the new biology. In C. P. Friedman & E. F. Purcell (Eds.), *The new biology and medical education: Merging the biological, information and cognitive sciences* (pp. 278–286). New York: Josiah Macy, Jr. Foundation.

Powles, A. C. P., Wintrup, N., Neufeld, V. R., Wakefield, J. H., Coates, G., & Burrows, J. (1981). The Triple Jump Exercise: Further studies of an evaluative technique. Research in medical education: 1981. *Proceedings of the 20th Annual Conference*. Washington, D.C.: American Association of Medical Colleges.

Williams, R. G., Vu, N. V., Barrows, H. G., & Verhulst, S. (1983). Profile of the Clinical Reasoning Test (CRT): An objective measure of problem solving skills and proficiency in using medical knowledge. In H. G. Schmidt & M. V. de Valdes (Eds.), *Tutorials on problem based learning*. Assen, The Netherlands: Van Gorcum.

Willoughby, T. L., & Hutcheson, S. J. (1978). Edumetric validity of the Quarterly Profile Examination. *Educational Psychology Measurement, 38*, 1057–1061.

Wingard, J. R., & Williamson, J. W. (1973). Grades as predictors of physicians' cover performance: An evaluative literature review. *Journal of Medical Education, 48*, 311.

CHAPTER 9

Admissions into a Problem-Based Curriculum

NANCY MARTINEZ-BURROLA,
DIANE J. KLEPPER, AND ARTHUR KAUFMAN

I think it is a fair statement . . . that an admissions committee consists of a group of medical school faculty members who are trying, with the best will in the world, to clone themselves. (Geiger, 1981, p. 42)

Goals

The medical school's admissions procedure should take account of the following:

1. Society's needs as well as an applicant's academic qualifications.
2. The applicant's predicted achievement of the school's ultimate educational goals, not simply short-term classroom performance.
3. An applicant's problem-solving skills, interpersonal skills, self-motivation, and level of maturity.
4. Predictors of an applicant's future practice specialty and location.

Introduction

There is a discordance between the traditional criteria for admissions into most medical schools and the ultimate goals of medical education. Such criteria are even more ill-suited to a problem-based curriculum. Major problems with medical school admissions are identified in the recently completed national survey of medical schools conducted by the Association of American Medical Colleges, entitled "Emerging Perspectives on the General Professional Education of the Physician" (GPEP, 1983). These problems include the following:

1. Despite a call for greater breadth in premedical education with greater emphasis on the social sciences and humanities, in reality, admissions committees still seem to overemphasize scientific preparation.
2. Reading, writing, and communication skills are basic to medicine yet sorely neglected in admissions criteria.
3. There is an overemphasis on the MCAT (Medical College Admissions Test) as an admissions criterion. It is inherently flawed in that it tends to evaluate test-taking ability rather than useful knowledge and bears no identifiable correlation with subsequent clinical performance.

Medical school admissions committees have traditionally selected students with the highest academic qualifications (grade point average, MCAT). These students tend to be male, white, urban, and middle- to upper-class (Elliot, 1975). This has become accentuated by the decline in student loans, and rise in school tuition, forcing even further reductions in applicants from blue-collar and rural families (Kiely, 1982). Currently, 48 percent of the places in medical school classes in the United States are occupied by students from families in the top 4 percent of the population by income. It is predicted that this economic force will reverse the current trend toward more physicians locating in underserved areas (Geiger, 1981).

While selection based primarily upon academic criteria may ensure a high level of student success in the first two years of medical school, it does not correlate with achievement in the clinical years (Schofield, 1970).

This raises questions about the role of such admissions variables in the selection of students for a problem-based curriculum. For in both problem-based tutorials and clinical rotations, students are judged primarily on how they identify, characterize, and solve problems, how they interact with peers and faculty, and how well they assume responsibility for their own learning. Since few grades and test scores comprising the traditional "academic record" assess these dimensions of the student's premedical performance, the admissions committee is left with little information upon which to judge the applicant on these very important qualities.

There is mounting evidence that medical school admissions criteria have impact beyond successful completion of medical school on future geographic choice and specialty practice (Cullison, Reid, & Colwill, 1976). And there is growing criticism that traditional admissions procedures select against students who would be more likely to later enter primary-care specialties and settle in underserved areas (Campbell, Rank, & Sinclair, 1974; Elliot, 1975; Geiger, 1981).

One factor having the most value in predicting those applicants most likely to later deliver primary care in underserved areas is demographic background. In a study of 1,146 graduates of the University of Missouri—Columbia Medical School, students from rural as opposed to urban backgrounds were found to be two to three times more likely to eventually practice in rural areas (Cullison et al., 1976). Another study found an increased likelihood of graduates selecting rural practice when the spouse came from a rural area (Taylor, Dickman, & Kane, 1973).

In what way have the problem-based medical school programs attempted to broaden student selection criteria to better match students to the unique needs of the curriculum and to choose students who will best fulfill perceived future needs in society?

University of New Mexico Program

The University of New Mexico School of Medicine is publicly supported and has two primary obligations. One is to offer state residents an opportunity to pursue a career in medicine, and the other is to train students who are likely to serve the state's health care needs. Residents of New Mexico, therefore, are given primary consideration for admission to the school. An active minority recruitment program encourages applications from New Mexico's Hispanic, Native American, and Black populations. The University is also a member of the Western Interstate Commission for Higher Education (WICHE). Consequently, special consideration is given to residents of the Western, rural states that have no medical schools—Alaska, Idaho, Montana, and Wyoming. Further, traditionally, an applicant's maturity, life experience, and interview score are heavily weighted so that, from 1979 to 1983, the composition of the student body has been 20 percent minorities, 35 percent women, 47.5 percent from rural backgrounds, and a freshman class averaging 25.5 years of age.

This orientation of the Medical School Admissions committee is so consonant with that of the PCC program that selection criteria into PCC are mostly fulfilled at the time of school acceptance. A PCC Admissions Subcommittee makes the final selection for each class. To streamline the subcommittee's work, until recently, the group was weighted with members from the main Medical School Admissions Committee who were familiar with the applicants' admissions folders.

Mindful of the growing concern about a predicted excess of physicians in the United States, PCC opted not to increase the total class size of 73 but increased the proportion of the fixed class size entering PCC; 10 the first year, 15 the second, and 20 each succeeding year. Thus, from its inception, the School of Medicine made a decision to reduce the number of conventionally prepared physicians to accommodate the experimental curriculum.

Also cognizant of a concern among some medical educators that "primary care" implies "less than" and that a program so oriented might serve as a "back door" into medical school for the less qualified, PCC planners decided to consider only applicants who had already gained acceptance to medical school. Those students desiring but not accepted into PCC matriculate in the conventional track. In this way, to become a student in the problem-based track or to express an early preference for rural primary care via the new track required more rigorous admissions hurdles. This was PCC's first political decision concerning admissions.

In the early years of the program preference was given to students from rural and medically underserved communities. Preference was also given to students demonstrating responsibility and work experience. In practice it was impossible for subcommittee members to reach a consensus about the appropriate weighting among these different variables.

To explore the relationship among these variables, PCC applicants' scores on the three separate scales—cognitive, noncognitive, and rural potential—were analyzed for the classes of 1985 and 1986. A Pearson's correlation coefficient was obtained on the data set of 52 subjects, and a significant negative relationship ($r = -.488, < .0001$) was found between cognitive rank and rural potential rank. The higher the rural potential rank, the lower the cognitive rank.

Recruiting

In the early years of the program there was considerable concern about whether enough admitted students would apply for PCC. How many students would risk their career on a totally untested track? Even PCC faculty could only speculate when asked hard questions such as, "Will PCC provide sufficient basic science instruction?" or "Will I be competitive for residency positions when I graduate from PCC?" An active recruiting campaign was begun with local newspaper articles about the program, letters to all students admitted to medical school, and active solicitation by PCC faculty of admitted students rumored to be considering the new program.

PCC had no model experiences at other schools from which to draw guidance. Most problem-based schools had only one track, and were thus "the only action in town." While Michigan State University had two tracks, they permitted students to experience elements of each over the first 10 weeks of school, thus giving the problem-based track time to "strut their stuff." At UNM, admitted students had to make a decision, sight-unseen, on the basis of faith.

Admitted students were given a fact-sheet in which PCC tried to lay out the program plan, address emerging misconceptions, and allay fears. That document was to undergo several revisions over the years as the program shifted emphasis and various concerns and rumors about the program emerged from applicants on admissions interviews. For example the introductory statement in the 1979 edition read:

> PCC is designed to increase the number of graduates entering primary care specialties (family practice, general internal medicine, general pediatrics) and locating in rural areas of the state.

This was later seen as one of the key barriers to students applying to PCC. Despite the impression left by the majority of applicants to UNM during their admissions interviews that their career plans were to become rural, primary-care physicians, much of this was intended simply to win favor with the interviewer. In fact, most applicants were uncertain about careers and few wanted to make such a commitment at the commencement of their medical education. Further, over the first five years of the program, PCC broadened its appeal, focusing more on educational methodology, less on practice site and specialization. It now viewed its rural, primary-care experiences not only in terms of career recruitment but as beneficial for the student's educational balance regardless of ultimate specialty choice. Thus the revised introductory statement in the 1983 edition of the information flyer read:

> PCC is a four-year curriculum track leading to the medical degree at the UNM School of Medicine. It is open to students interested in all fields of

medicine (research, primary care, subspecialties) and offers broad exposure in each. The uniqueness of PCC lies in its educational philosophy and methods.

Selecting/Rejecting

The final criterion for selection into PCC changed each year as the subcommittee responded to external forces. Since the initial stated goals of the program emphasized underserved, rural practice, applicants in the first two classes showing strong promise in these areas were both recruited and favored over applicants weaker in these areas but with stronger cognitive scores. After a disastrous National Board performance by the second PCC class, it was clear that many long-term goals would have to be deferred to first build faculty acceptance of the new educational method—a short-term goal. Thus, over the five years, cognitive abilities grew as a weighting factor in the selection process.

As PCC moved to broaden the appeal of the program, students with interests in all fields, including academia and research, were encouraged to apply. No longer would an applicant's inability to relocate away from Albuquerque for a rural preceptorship (Chapter 7) preclude further consideration. For such students the program would accommodate the student by establishing sites within commuting distance of Albuquerque.

Because each year there were five to ten unsuccessful applicants to PCC in the conventional track, PCC planners were concerned about the lingering resentment against PCC of students in this group. Some of these PCC rejectees were embittered. Several had wanted admission to PCC as much as to medical school itself. For them, the experiment was creating anxiety and resentment more than educational options.

Admissions Procedure:
First Step in a Study Design

Fortuitously, by narrowing the PCC applicant pool to already admitted students and fixing the ceiling at a limit of 20 PCC slots per class, the admissions process lent itself well to a subsequent study design of the program (Chapter 10). The number of applicants to PCC gradually increased over the first 6 years, growing from 16 (22% of the admitted class) the first year to 34 (47%) the sixth.

Initially it was decided that students applying to and acceptable to PCC would be randomized into PCC and the conventional track, thus permitting an identified control group. This was quickly thwarted after the first year owing to short-term political goals cited above and a concern that the number of applicants randomized into the conventional program would be few, making later statistical comparison between tracks extremely difficult.

Thus, for four years, each student in the admitted PCC class was matched with a conventional-track student on the basis of MCATs, grade-point average, sex, ethnicity, and age. This group served as a match control, ostensibly differing only in that they had preferred the conventional program upon admission to medical school. This assumption, it was later learned, was inaccurate. Many research-wise critics felt that with the current study design one could not distinguish which program outcomes were attributable to the PCC curriculum and which to students' self-selection.

Thus, by the fifth year, after considerable acceptance and institutionalization of PCC within the medical school, program planners felt secure enough to once again randomize acceptable applicants into PCC and the conventional program (Figure 9.1). Though the numbers randomized into the conventional program might be small each year, it was hoped that growth of the applicant pool and a consistent study design would eventuate in a sizable number in this group over the years.

Figure 9.1.   Revised admissions procedure. First step in a study design. (Assume that 30 students request experimental track.)

ACCEPTED: 73 **(APPLIED:** Approx. 300)	30 Request experimental track	20 Accepted into experimental track	Experimental group
		10 Randomized out of experimental into conventional track	Randomized controls
	43 Request conventional track	20 in conventional track matched with experimental group	Matched controls
		23 in conventional track, nonrandomized, nonmatched	Nonrandomized nonmatched controls

Program planners believed that another benefit of this new admissions procedure and study design would be that unsuccessful applicants to PCC would not have to feel that they were "rejected" or "unacceptable"—they knew the computer merely randomized them into the conventional track. This was a gross error in judgment, for the program merely traded one necessary evil for another.

Many students now resented being randomized by a computer rather than chosen for PCC on their merits:

> *"I really want to demonstrate to you why I'm right for PCC, how I can really bring something special to the program. And now I'm not even being given the chance. It just galls me that another student I know is applying and doesn't really care that much which track she's in. Now she's got as much chance to get into PCC as I do."*

Who Applies to PCC?

Over the past five years (1979–1983) a total of 364 students matriculated into the UNM School of Medicine. Of those, 118 chose to apply to PCC. This pool of applicants differed from students choosing the conventional track in a number of respects.

Students selecting PCC scored significantly lower on the chemistry and physics portions of the Medical College Admissions Test (Table 9.1). Their mean grade-point average (overall, science, and nonscience) was also lower (Table 9.2).

All applicants to UNM School of Medicine receive two interviews. Between 1981 and 1983 one interview was "blinded" (interviewer has

Table 9.1. Comparison of MCAT Scores between Applicants to the PCC and Conventional Tracks (Two-Sample t-Test)

	PCC	Conventional	p-value
Number of applicants (n)	$n = 118$	$n = 246$	
Biology	9.07	9.30	n.s.
Chemistry	8.83	9.27	$<.05$
Physics	8.51	9.08	$<.05$
Sciences problems	8.89	9.29	n.s.
Reading comprehension	9.07	8.95	n.s.
Quantitative	8.71	8.75	n.s.

Table 9.2. Comparison of Grade-Point Averages between Applicants to the PCC and Conventional Tracks (Two-Sample *t*-Test)

	PCC	Conventional	p-value
Number of applicants (n)	n = 118	n = 245	
Overall GPA	3.26	3.43	<.001
Science GPA	3.21	3.41	<.001
Nonscience GPA	3.34	3.46	< .01

no prior information about the applicant) and one was "sighted" (interviewer has full access to the applicant's cognitive scores and admissions folder). Interviewers wrote a narrative assessment on each applicant and ranked the applicant on seven noncognitive dimensions using a seven-point scale. An overall score was also assigned.

While it has been found that overall ratings were similar between the "blinded" and "sighted" interviewers, "blinded" interviewers rated applicants significantly higher in the dimensions of motivation, background, and maturity ($p < .05$). In a comparison of noncognitive scores for applicants who subsequently applied to PCC with those subsequently applying to the conventional track, PCC applicants had received significantly higher scores from "blinded" interviewers in the dimensions of problem-solving, motivation, and maturity. ($p < .05$).

Age comparison between applicants to PCC ($\bar{x} = 25.7$) and conventional track ($\bar{x} = 23.4$) showed the former to be significantly older ($p < .0001$). No significant differences appeared in the sex, urban versus rural background, or ethnicity of applicants (Table 9.3).

Table 9.3. Comparison of Demographic Variables between Applicants to the PCC and Conventional Tracks (Chi-Square Analysis)

Variables	PCC Applicants	Conventional Applicants	Probability
	n=118	n=246	
Females	41%	33%	n.s.
Rural background	53%	45%	n.s.
Minority status	27%	22%	n.s.

PCC's emphasis on early assumption of responsibility for learning on the part of its students may have played a large part in the attractiveness of PCC to older students. PCC's environment was more consonent with the degree of control over their lives to which older students had become accustomed. Most stated that it was difficult to contemplate once again returning to the constraints of a lecture hall. Older students were more likely to have families and preferred PCC's more flexible schedule.

Why Students Select Each Track

Each year, after admissions decisions are completed, students within each track are sampled to determine the reasons for their choice of track. The great majority of students who applied to PCC did so for its educational approach and supportive environment.

> *"I am an older student and was attracted to PCC because I felt it would be easier on my family, less pressure, more interaction, and a better learning style for my needs."*

> *"I chose to come to the New Mexico School of Medicine because of PCC—I would have been very discouraged if I hadn't gotten in the track. . . . It is the first time I have been in a nonpunitive educational system. I used to rebel against my early schooling, but PCC is a program that respects its students."*

> *"I only applied to the UNM Medical School because of PCC. I had known about the program since it began in 1979. I was so committed to its educational philosophy that I probably would have reconsidered going to med school had I not gotten into PCC."*

> *"I knew I could make it in the regular track. It was just like all undergraduate courses. PCC posed a challenge for me."*

For some students PCC resembled positive experiences they had had in the past.

> *"I experienced a similar setup at St. John's College and so was drawn to PCC's unstructured aspects. I find lecture-learning too passive and don't believe in memorizing massive amounts of material. I like setting my own learning goals."*

> *"I chose PCC because it was very similar to the learning environment I experienced while doing research."*

And some students were ambivalent about their choice:

> *"I was ambivalent at first. I had poor study habits and tended to learn well for tests but then forget the material. On the other hand, I felt PCC offered the motivation for learning from peers instead of from exams. I finally chose PCC."*

Most students choosing the conventional track favored its familiar method of teaching and learning.

> *"The regular track offers the normal way of learning."*

> *"Ever since hearing about PCC from the Pre-Med Club I knew I would choose the regular track. I was never really good at self-study—I do better with lectures and outlines of what is expected. I guess I wasn't motivated enough for PCC."*

> *"I went into the regular track because I wanted a solid basic science background. I will be spending the rest of my life doing the clinical side of medicine."*

Some students saw PCC as limiting—a preparation only for rural or primary care. Others found the idea of relocating for the rural preceptorship too great a personal hardship.

Response of UNM Medical School
Faculty to PCC Admissions
Procedures

Response of faculty not centrally involved in PCC concerning the criteria of admissions into the program has been varied and vocal. Those most remote from the program felt that PCC should be an option only for the most mature, independent-minded, motivated, and scientifically prepared students. They felt that the curricular structure was so loose and evaluation methods so impressionistic that weak students or those unaccustomed to such freedom and responsibility would flounder and their acquisition of scientific content would be spotty. Thus, considerable pressure was put on the PCC admissions subcommittee to exclude from consideration "high-risk" students.

Years of experience showed that PCC's image within the medical school was very much a creature of faculty's first impressions. Thus, if PCC accepted many academically high-risk students who subsequently performed poorly on National Boards, faculty external to the program would tend to attribute the students' test performances to the PCC curriculum, not to their premedical preparation and test-taking ability. Despite the lack of data supporting the contention that high-risk students did any worse in PCC, and some evidence to the contrary (see Chapter 10), this climate of faculty concern led to a politically motivated decision on the part of PCC planners to compromise and eliminate from consideration students whose cognitive scores made them "very" high risk.

Disappointing to PCC at first, though understandable, was the very cautious attitude toward PCC of the Minority Affairs Office in the medical school. With 20 to 25 percent of the admitted students minority, it was hoped by PCC planners that a strong alliance could be forged with this office, which was so influential in recruiting and advising minority applicants to the medical school. Though roughly an equal proportion of admitted minorities applied to PCC as applied to the conventional track, PCC expected a much higher percentage in light of the academically supportive, socially cooperative, self-paced nature of the experimental track. However, some minority office representatives expressed the concern that weaker minority students may need more academic structure. Over the years PCC has come to rely on the expertise of this office for minority recruitment and retention. They currently guide those students toward PCC who they think will be successful and are prompt in offering supportive interaction when PCC asks for their assistance.

In the minds of some faculty the medical school admissions committee was relying too heavily on the "soft," subjective interview impressions and noncognitive data, and too lightly upon the "hard," objective, numerical data of applicants' MCATs and grades. For some, "soft" was equated with "PCC" and when several applicants with weaker cognitive scores openly stated their preferences for the experimental track during admissions interviews and were subsequently admitted, a howl went up in certain quarters that applicants desiring PCC were receiving special consideration. Thus, to remove the impression that certain applicants were being admitted to medical school because they expressed an interest in PCC, it was recommended that interviewers no longer inquire about applicants' track preference. Also, to remove any stigma of conflict of interest, it was agreed that members of the PCC Admissions Subcommittee would not also serve on the general medical school Admissions Committee.

What We Have Learned

1. Prospective applicants should be presented with clearly defined goals and methods of the new curriculum as well as applicant qualities deemed suitable for such a curriculum. Such information must be broadly advertised to all potential

applicants. Since the student chooses the program, it is imperative that misinformation be minimized and the choices clarified.

2. It is important to identify which applicant evaluation variables are best suited to each program goal. It may be necessary to develop and test new admissions screening instruments if available ones seem unsuitable.

3. Admissions criteria should weigh noncognitive variables heavily, for premedical cognitive scores are predictive of medical school test scores only in the first two years of a traditional program and are even less predictive of performance in problem-based tutorials.

4. Admissions decisions can have enormous political implications. During early program implementation, decisions about applicants may have to serve short-term political interests to spare long-term program goals.

5. The admissions process can be an important first step in an educational research design to evaluate the program outcomes.

Experience at Other Schools

Michigan State University (MSU) has run a problem-based curriculum track for the first two years of medical school since 1973 (Echt & Chan, 1977). Like the New Mexico program, it accepts students only after their admission to the medical school. However, students at MSU make their preference after all students have completed a ten-week introductory phase offering experiences in both teacher-centered and student-centered learning environments. All students selecting the problem-based option ("Track II") are accepted into that track.

The MSU admission design offers two advantages. First, students are able to make a more informed choice. In the New Mexico program the choice is made without the hindsight of experience, and many students later feel cheated that they were not sufficiently informed before selection. Printed material is simply an inadequate basis upon which to make such an important curricular track decision. Second, by admitting all interested medical students into Track II, the lingering bitterness of rejected applicants within the conventional program is obviated. In New Mexico, applicants rejected because of either randomization or insufficient qualifications create an undercurrent of dissatisfaction as the school year begins.

The disadvantage of the MSU method of admission in a two-track medical school is its deleterious effect on a clean study design. One cannot easily distinguish subsequent program outcomes of the problem-based track from the unique qualities of the students who have self-selected into that curriculum. Thus, in a two-track program, the ability to institute some form of randomization at the time of admission offers important opportunities to study the effect of the curriculum upon its students. Schools that are solely problem-based, such as McMaster, Mercer, Maastricht, and Newcastle obviously cannot conduct such a study design within their schools. However, randomization in the admissions has now been instituted into the problem-based track within the Introduction to Clinical Medicine course at the University of Colorado.

McMaster University has experimented with an innovative approach to screening and selecting applicants for their problem-based tutorial curriculum. Their admissions committee was concerned that college grades, recommendation letters, and personal interviews did not provide sufficient information about an applicant's capacity to handle problems or work productively and cooperatively within a group. The committee thus constructed an admissions exercise in which applicants would be observed working in the same manner expected of them in the problem-based curriculum. Students were randomly assigned to work on problems in tutorial groups (Ferrier, McAuley, & Roberts 1978; Mitchell, Pallie, & McAuley, 1975). The "admissions" tutorial exercise was observed through a one-way mirror, and each applicant's performance was rated on terms of approach to the problem and interpersonal skills. Evaluation of the simulated tutorial at McMaster showed that the exercise was both feasible and tended to predict how applicants subsequently functioned in small educational groups.

The planners of the program at Ben-Gurion University of the Negev at Beersheba, Israel, addressing a different set of program goals than those at MSU and McMaster, developed different criteria for admission. The Ben-Gurion orientation is toward primary care and community medicine. To be fully effective in such a setting, the physician must work effectively on a health care team, emphasize disease prevention, and be capable of working effectively with various ethnic, socioeconomic, and religious population subgroups. Thus the Ben-Gurion admissions procedure both advertises and emphasizes emotional and intellectual characteristics in applicants most compatible with these goals (Antonovsky, 1976).

To emphasize this point, above a minimum grade-point average applicants gain no advantage for having earned higher grades. Further, in the Beersheba program there is no advantage to having majored in one field of study over another. A degree in the humanities is equivalent to one in the sciences. Older candidates are clearly favored for "we felt that candidates whose total life experience was largely limited to the school desk were not for us" (Antonovsky, 1976, p. 4). Though not a stated policy of PCC admissions, the New Mexico program also attracts and selects students who are, on the average, three years older than their conventional-track peers.

Implications

The likelihood of a medical school dramatically altering its admissions procedures is enhanced if innovation characterizes other important aspects of the medical school program. Major modifications in curricular design and teaching strategies exerts pressure on the admissions process to better select students for the new educational environment.

A problem-based, tutorial learning program, in particular, creates considerable demands for a selection process that values an applicant's interactive skills, level of maturity, and responsibility, for these qualities are both visible and challenged from the beginning of medical school. In a conventional, didactic curriculum, on the other hand, academic achievement alone may suffice as a predictor of student performance during the first two years. Most academic failures surface during these early years, and student deficiencies in the later, clinical years are poorly identified in most medical schools. Thus, in a conventional curriculum, a faculty can be lulled into a false sense of security when it is satisfied that its admissions emphasis on academic achievement predicts "student success." It is likely that our schools have simply done little to evaluate which admissions criteria correlate with later clinical performance.

The need for experimentation in medical school admissions is both timely and critical. The new problem-based medical school programs have provided an important impetus for such long-neglected studies.

References

Antonovsky, A. (1976). Student selection in the School of Medicine, Ben-Gurion University of the Negev. *Medical Education, 10,* 219–234.

Campbell, E. F., Rank, B. K., & Sinclair, A. J. M. (1974). Selection of medical students—A burning question. *Medical Journal of Australia, 1,* 785–788.

Cullison, S., Reid, C., & Colwill, J. M. (1976). Medical school admissions specialty selection and distribution of physicians. *Journal of the American Medical Association, 235,* 502–505.

Echt, R., & Chan, S. (1977). A new problem-oriented and student-centered curriculum at Michigan State University. *Journal of Medical Education, 52,* 681–683.

Elliot, P. R. (1975, May). *The admissions process: How to select for the family practice student.* Paper presented to Second Annual Conference on Undergraduate Education in Family Practice, Kansas City, Mo.

Emerging perspectives on the general professional education of the physician. (1983, October). Washington, D.C.: American Association of Medical Colleges.

Ferrier, B. M., McAuley, R. G., & Roberts, R. S. (1978). Selection of medical students at McMaster University. *Journal of the Royal College of Physicians, 12,* 365–378.

Geiger, H. J. (1981). Affirmative action in medical school admissions. In *Troubling problems in medical ethics* (Vol. 3, pp. 39–45). New York: Alan R. Liss Inc.

Kiely, J. M. (1982). Editorial, medical school admissions: Winds of change. *Mayo Clinic Proceedings, 57,* 598–599.

Mitchell, D. L. M., Pallie, W., & McAuley, R. G. (1975). The simulated tutorial: Method for assessing medical students' applicants. *British Journal of Medical Education, 9,* 133–139.

Schofield, W. (1970). A modified actuarial method in the selection of medical students. *Journal of Medical Education, 45,* 740–744.

Taylor, M., Dickman, W., and Kane, R. (1973). Medical students' attitudes toward rural practice. *Journal of Medical Education, 48,* 885–895.

CHAPTER 10

Program Evaluation

MAGGI MOORE-WEST AND MICHAEL J. O'DONNELL

Only rarely do we find experimental or quasi-experimental research designs to test whether an innovation has attained its intended goals. (Howell, 1979, p. 169)

Design of Evaluation

PCC was evaluated to assess the program primarily in the following four areas: (1) students' academic performance, (2) students' career orientation, (3) students' attitudes, and (4) faculty's attitudes. The coexistence of a conventional track and a problem-based track were a fortunate circumstance at the University of New Mexico School of Medicine (UNM-SOM) because it provided the framework for an ideal investigation. PCC exploited this dual track opportunity by designing a prospective, longitudinal study in which the experimental PCC group was matched with conventional-track control groups housed on the same campus (see Chapter 9).

At the PCC program's outset a prospective, longitudinal study attempted to answer four questions:

1. Are there differences in personality profile and demographic background between students choosing the problem-based and conventional tracks?
2. Are there differences in the effect of problem-based versus conventional education on the quality of the students' learning?

3. Can the curriculum influence the students' career orientation and practice location?

4. Can the differences between the curricula cause differences in the students' attitudes toward medical education, levels of confidence and self-esteem, and perceived stress?

Table 10.1 presents a sample schedule of selected scales, question-naires, and tests administered by the Longitudinal Study group. This is a team of evaluators studying the development and results of the problem-based curriculum within the context of the medical school. Students in both tracks as well as faculty are subjects of the studies. Instruments and their administration schedules have varied over the years in response to early study results and changing program needs.

Students were followed throughout their four years of medical school by the use of scales and questionnaires, interviews, observations, and group meetings. Owing to logistical constraints, data on third-year students is gathered through individual and group interviews and through observations of ward behavior. Fourth-year students are given an exit interview eliciting an assessment of their medical education and factors influencing their career choice. Finally, faculty who have tutored PCC students or supervised their hospital ward work completed a questionnaire concerning attitudes toward problem-based versus conventional education.

The chapter will sumarize some of the initial findings of our attempts to answer the above questions.

Personality Variables

The characteristics of students applying to and entering PCC compared to those in the conventional track differed in some respects (see Chapter 9). In an attempt to determine whether personality influences self-selection into and ultimate success in each track, various instruments assessing personality profiles and traits were administered to students upon entry into medical school (e.g., Myers-Briggs Personality Type Inventory, Kolb's Learning Style, Embedded Figures Test, California Psychological Inventory). The results of the Myers-Briggs Personality Type Inventory (MBPTI) will be reported here because the test incorporates many features of the other instruments. Further, it is widely used in medical education research, is easily administered, and takes only about 35 minutes to complete; moreover feedback to individual students about their profile is easily given.*

*MBPTI can be purchased from Consulting Psychologist's Press, Inc., 577 College Ave., Palo Alto, CA 94306, (415)847–1447.

Table 10.1. Sample Schedule of Scales, Questionnaires, and Tests Administered to Students and Faculty by the Longitudinal Study Program of the University of New Mexico

	Dates of Administration					
Items Studied	Orientation	2nd Semester	3rd Semester	4th Semester	3rd Year	4th Year
I. Students						
A. Demographic information	X					
B. Personality profiles	X					
C. Academic performance						
1. NBME-I				X		
2. Ward performance					X	
D. Career preference	X					X
E. Student attitudes						
1. Symptoms questionnaire	X	X	X	X		
2. Attitudes toward basic sciences	X	X	X	X		
II. Faculty						
F. Faculty attitudes			(Variable)			

The MBPTI bears some relationship with specialty choice, academic achievement, and performance on some standardized objective examinations (McCaully, 1977). It is an instrument designed to categorize individuals based on the way they perceive and make judgments about the world around them. It measures four dimensions of a person's cognitive and perceptual style.

1. *Extroversion/introversion* indicates whether one is apt to "act on the world" or be more reflective.
2. *Sensing/intuition* measures whether one perceives through the senses and is attuned to detail, or perceives through imagination and reviews many possibilities.
3. *Thinking/feeling* indicates whether one makes decisions based on logic or based on feelings about the situation.
4. *Judging/perceptive* measures whether one is quick to make judgments and maintain them, or waits until more information is available.

The MBPTI was administered during orientation to each study group in the classes of 1983 to 1985 and to the entire student body since the class of 1986. Data on the first five classes were combined for purposes of comparison.

Outcomes on the first administration of the MBPTI revealed significant differences (Table 10.2). A greater number of "extroverted, intuitive, feeling" individuals appeared in the PCC group; "introverted, sensing, and thinking" in the conventional group.

To determine whether personality type influenced performance on the National Board of Medical Examiners Part I (NBME-I), available data were analyzed on students having previously taken the MBPTI for purposes of Board preparation. Success on NBME-I was determined for 74 students who fit into either extreme of the MBPTI: the "Sensing-Thinking-Judging" (STJ) group, which prefers logic, facts, and decisiveness, and the "Intuitive-Feeling-Perceptive" (NFP) group, which prefers ideas, feelings, and options. While a higher percentage of NFPs in the conventional track group failed Boards (25 of 44 = 57 percent) than did NFPs in PCC (4 of 16 = 25 percent), the numbers were small and the differences not significant. While no STJs failed Boards in the conventional track, there were no STJs in the PCC sample against which to compare. More data will be collected to determine whether there are significant correlations between particular personality types and Board performance.

Initial differences between MBPTI scores of students applying to PCC versus the conventional track suggest that self-selection is an

Table 10.2.   Comparison of PCC and Conventional Match Students on Myers-Briggs Personality Inventory, Combining Classes 1983–1987

	Myers-Briggs Personality Inventory		
	Extrovert	Introvert	Chi Square Complex
PCC (*n* = 85)	51	34	
Conventional matched (*n* = 78)	26	57	*p*<.007
	Intuitive	Sensing	
PCC (*n* = 85)	67	18	
Conventional matched (*n* = 78)	39	39	*p*<.0001
	Feeling	Thinking	
PCC (*n* = 85)	54	31	
Conventional matched (*n* = 78)	34	44	*p*<.01
	Judging	Perceptive	
PCC (*n* = 85)	43	42	
Conventional matched (*n* = 78)	29	49	N.S.

important entry variable to be followed in studying subsequent student performance. It appears that students preferring PCC were those who were more attracted to the stimulation of new ideas, to rebelling against tradition. They saw the conventional curriculum as "intolerable," and they were disdainful of traditional test-taking procedures.

Conversely, the personality of students preferring the conventional curriculum supported a skepticism about trusting their futures to a method that had not been tested. Without guidance, they were uncomfortable in their ability to select what was important to learn, and they were concerned about the ambiguity of the PCC methods.

These findings have important implications for medical educators and curriculum planners. PCC is an experimental curriculum which requires students to manage their own learning. Since they are challenged to contend with many interpersonal demands, and since ambiguity within the program is high, skills in interpersonal communication and adaptability are essential. Thus it is understandable that students with these personality traits would be attracted to PCC.

For more sensing, introverted students, the conventional track's lecture format might be more attractive because of its formal routine, its attention to detail, and its more impersonal approach. As the traditional method of teaching, it is more attractive to students preferring the tried and true. Introverted and sensing-type students also may shy away from ambiguous circumstances and might avoid a new program which is student-centered and which requires a high level of adaptability. It appears that students with certain personality traits tend to choose a curriculum compatible with that personality's learning style. Whether such a match eventuates in a measurable improvement in student learning requires further investigation.

A question arises as to whether the type of student who chooses the PCC curriculum is the type of student who will likely fulfill its goals. An orientation to rural primary care is one such goal. Previous research of MBPTI and career choices (McCaully, 1977) has indicated that the more introverted, sensing type, who is dependable, practical, and interested in working with people will be the type preferring a rural locale. The extroverted, intuitive type, on the other hand, is good at generating new ideas and solving problems, but might become bored if rural practice were to become a routine. Students of this latter type may find stimulation and excitement in the rural communities, yet their roles might differ from the current norm. Instead, these physicians may move to a community for a limited time, identify health care needs, and develop programs to meet those needs, rather than provide direct long-term clinical services.

National Boards and Clinical Performance

National Board of
Medical Examiners
(NBME)

For many faculty the most critical evaluation of PCC was the students' performance on NBME Part I, given at the end of the second year. Passage of the examination is mandatory for promotion in each track. Since there are scant cognitive evaluations comparing the two tracks of students before this time, considerable interest was generated in Board performance for the first several classes of PCC students.

This presented PCC program planners with an opportunity and a dilemma. If students in the experimental track performed comparably to conventional-track students, much faculty concern about the students' ability to learn scientific information in such a loosely structured program would be allayed. But PCC valued an integration of clinical as well as basic sciences and emphasized the process of learning rather than the retention of content. It was therefore feared that the program would be unfairly judged by its students' performance on a pure, basic-science, memory-based content examination. Only time could tell.

There has been no significant difference between PCC vs. Match in performance on NBME Part I or Part II in terms of total scores (Figure 10.1). Yet, in the early years members of PCC experienced a roller coaster of emotions with each test result. The first PCC class took NBME-I in 1981. They performed significantly lower only in the anatomy subsection of the examination. For a first outing, results for the

Figure 10.1. NBME Part I and NBME Part II total scores of graduating classes 1983–1985 PCC vs. Match.*

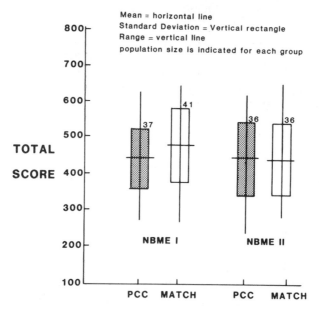

* There are no significant differences in total scores between PCC and Match groups either on NBME parts I or II. Part I scores = highest score achieved on either June or September administration at end of second year.

first class of PCC students were generally acceptable. Students could accumulate sufficient content in a loosely structured, problem-based curriculum to pass a national, standardized examination. The program's response: stay the course.

The second class of PCC students presented the program with a challenge. As a class, they had begun to express anxiety about NBME-I at the beginning of medical school. The program had paid little attention to their anxiety and provided little structured preparation for NBME-I.

When July 1982 came, the Board results stunned the PCC faculty and students. Six passed and six failed. In the matched control group, 9 passed and 3 failed. Comparison between PCC and the matched group showed PCC students had now scored significantly lower on the Anatomy and Physiology sections of the examination.

But closer examination of the results revealed less disparity between the two tracks than originally thought. With "high risk" defined by MCAT scores of 48 and under, three of the conventional match students who failed Boards were high risk compared to four of the PCC students (Table 10.3).

Concern grew about the academic caliber and test-taking ability of the students attracted to PCC. As a result, PCC instituted a more stringent selection policy. While there had been an initial pressure from some research-minded faculty to randomize all interested PCC applicants into both tracks, a growing number of faculty now protested against considering applicants to PCC who had low MCAT and GPA scores. The program made a compromise. Students with lower cognitive scores would be scrutinized more carefully before inclusion in the pool from which the PCC class would be chosen. But many in PCC seriously questioned the rationale for this decision, fearing that the program was overreacting to one group of low scores and, perhaps, sacrificing a more

Table 10.3. Comparison of NBME-I Results in Relation to MCAT Performance between Tracks for Class of 1984

	PCC			Conventional Matched		
MCAT Scores	Passed	Failed		MCAT Scores	Passed	Failed
>49	5	2		>49	7	0
<48	2	4		<48	2	3

important goal of selecting some students who would most likely turn to rural or underserved areas. There was further concern that Boards may not be adequate predictors of clinical performance, and therefore an altered admissions policy might select against students who would perform better clinically. By narrowing the field of acceptable applicants, PCC's ability to determine the effects of problem-based, tutorial learning on students from varied backgrounds and skill levels would be curtailed.

Greater emphasis was now placed on preparing and counseling students about NBME-I. With the introduction of NBME-I seven subject Shelf Boards (Chapter 8) administered twice yearly, PCC had the opportunity to follow a student's test performance over two years. Evaluators identified and encouraged academically weak students in the class of 1985 to wait until September to take NBME-I to allow them adequate preparation time. The class of 1985 performed well on NBME-I, and their scores returned to a level of comparability with the conventional-track students.

Ward Performance

All clinical rotations were analyzed for the classes of 1983 and 1984; two-thirds of the rotations of the class of 1985 could be analyzed by the time of submission of this manuscript. Prior to the class of 1985, the method of reporting student evaluations varied with departments but generally were translated into grades of "superior" (SUP), "satisfactory-plus" (SAT+), "satisfactory" (SAT), "satisfactory-minus" (SAT–), and "Unsatisfactory" (UNSAT).

The departments of psychiatry, surgery, and internal medicine were the only ones consistent in distinguishing between an overall grade and a clinical performance grade. Reporting of oral and written examinations varied in format between the departments, but their relative contribution to the overall grade could be inferred by any discrepancy between the overall and clinical grades.

A new, uniform grading policy was introduced beginning with the class of 1985. Different components of student performance on each rotation could now be compared because of the new, itemized evaluation forms. However, for purposes of consistency, we have analyzed only student performance on the same three rotations, measuring only the overall and clinical grades available for the prior two classes.

Figure 10.2 summarizes the combined ward performance of PCC and Matched Control Students in each of three rotations: psychiatry, surgery, and internal medicine. "Overall" and "clinical" ratings are

Figure 10.2. Performance of third-year clinical rotations for PCC and matched control students for classes of 1983, 1984, and 1985.

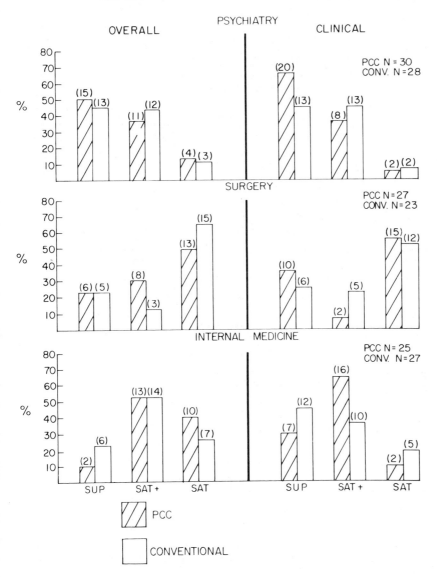

summarized separately. Results from a chi square analysis showed no significant differences in overall or clinical performance between students in each track.

Career Preference

Research has found that medical students show increasing interest in specialization as they progress through medical school (Rezler, 1974). Since there is traditional dominance of specialty role modeling in the University Hospital, it was important to determine whether PCC students' sustained rural, primary-care preceptorships and community-based electives would influence their career preferences. Such preferences were assessed at entry into medical school and after their residency match in their senior year. Because only two PCC classes have completed medical school, the data reported here were gathered for the classes of 1983 and 1984. Nineteen PCC students were compared to 19 conventional matched students.

Family practice is the most popular specialty preference for both groups at orientation (Figure 10.3). To test whether this interest is equally sustained for both tracks by graduation, a chi square for goodness of fit was performed. The results showed that by graduation the distribution of career preferences for PCC students remained essentially unchanged (Figure 10.4). For the conventional-track students the distribution of career preferences at graduation was significantly different. Internal medicine now became the preferred specialty for this group ($p < .005$).

Selecting Primary Care

If this trend is sustained, it will require further analysis. Do PCC students sustain their interest in family practice because of extensive contact with family practice physicians during their first two years? And since a majority of internists enter subspecialties (e.g., cardiology, hematology, rheumatology) in larger cities in which they practice little primary care, will differences in primary-care practice emerge between the study groups over time?

Of the 19 PCC graduates, eight have matched at UNM residencies (four—family practice, two—pediatrics, one—internal medicine, one—surgery). Their comparative performance at the residency level will be followed closely by a number of departments.

Figure 10.3. Comparison of PCC vs. conventional matched students on career preference during orientation (classes of 1983 and 1984).

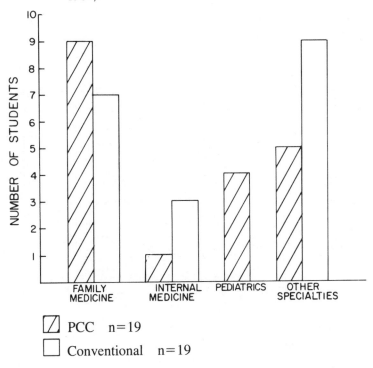

PCC n=19
Conventional n=19

Student Attitudes

Another type of study involves the nature of the experience that students undergo in PCC. This includes both an understanding of students' attitudes toward their environment and a description of the environment itself. Would PCC, with its student-centered learning and close, informal, student–faculty relationships, result in different student attitudes than a program where students attend lectures and predominantly respond to a faculty-directed curriculum?

Two of the scales chosen to monitor students' attitudes look at the issue from different perspectives: students' general emotional feelings, and students' attitudes toward basic sciences. The latter were measured because of a concern that students in such a clinically oriented track as PCC would see less value in basic science education.

Figure 10.4.   Comparison of PCC vs. conventional matched students on final
residency selection (classes of 1983 and 1984).

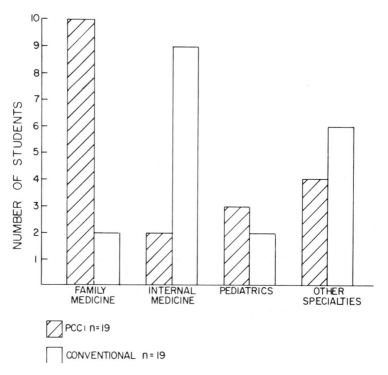

To measure general emotional feelings, students completed a
Symptom Questionnaire (SQ) designed by Kellner and Sheffield (1973)
to measure different dimensions of distress, somatic complaints, hostility, and anxiety. The sum of the four subscale scores is the Total Distress
Score and provides a measure of stress. The scale has been tested for
reliability and validity and has been frequently used in studies of
psychoactive drugs. With the exception of the classes of 1983 and 1987,
students were administered the questionnaire every semester for the first
two years. *T*–Tests were employed for significant differences between
PCC and the conventional track on each administration. It was hypothesized that stress would grow over time, in response to an intense, often
ambiguous, learning environment.

The average distress scores over the first two years of medical
school showed that PCC students perceived significantly less distress
than students in the matched track (as tested by an analysis of variance
with one repeated factor), despite the fact that both groups entered

medical school with similar stress scores ($\bar{x} = 13.94$ and $\bar{x} = 15.00$, for PCC and Match, respectively). (See Table 10.4.) Because of the difference in sample size between PCC and Matched tracks, we were concerned that there was a change in the distribution of matching variables that may have influenced these findings. However, a comparison of these two tracks on three of the important matching variables showed no difference between tracks in MCATs, gender, or ethnicity.

Students' attitudes toward basic sciences were measured by a scale modified from the Physician Ideology Questionnaire and the Student–Faculty Role Questionnaire (Otis & Weiss, 1972, 1973). Items were chosen that reflected the students' appreciation of basic science information, as well as the perceived value of their learning experiences within medical school. Results showed that students in the conventional track generally viewed the role of basic sciences as important, yet when faced with the need to learn "facts" separated from their clinical application, for many, the consequent tedium and need for memorization fostered a cynicism about how they were learning (West et al., 1982). This was not the case for PCC students who felt that what they were learning was relevant to their future roles.

Analysis of Student Attitudes

Observations and interviews from the comparisons of the two tracks indicate that the tracks differed in terms of stress levels and students' perception of their learning environment. As a group, students in the conventional track exhibited more stress than students in PCC. As one conventional-track student explained:

> *"At this point [second semester] I feel so burned out on medical school, medicine, and myself. My mind refuses to absorb any more*

Table 10.4. Means and Standard Deviations of Total Distress Scores for Kellner's Symptom Questionnaire*

	Mean	Standard Deviation	N
PCC	16.41	(8.41)	32
Match	27.57	(15.61)	19

*Medical school track (*PCC* versus *Match*) accounts for a significant 13% of the variance in total scores $F(1,34) = 6.85$, $p < .01$.

facts, and yet the faculty keep pumping them out to me, day in and day out. I feel so bad at times, to realize that I'm not studying to become a doctor, just to pass tests."

"I believe I've actually lost my ability to think. All I do is memorize facts to pass an exam. I think I'm losing sight of ever becoming a physician. And when you have the faculty standing up there and telling you what an idiot you are for not passing their exams, I sometimes wonder."

That there was significantly less stress among the PCC students is ironic given the amount of ambiguity in the experimental program and the increasing pressure from NBME-I for which there had not been the type of preparation that there was in the conventional program. In many ways their stress is different:

"Sometimes I hate being in this fishbowl. Especially when you have a faculty member approach you and tell you that you have to perform better than students in the conventional track in order for PCC to succeed. That's a lot of pressure. Yet I realize just how important PCC is to me. I could never imagine PCC faculty putting pressure on us like they do in the other track. I don't think I could have survived the alienation I see in students in the conventional curriculum."

For some students small groups can breed excessive scrutiny and pigeon-holing of individuals.

"PCC students are labeled and that label carries with them through the [first] two years of medical school. 'Good' students can do no wrong. But no one will listen to 'poor' students in the tutorial or take what they say seriously."

PCC students' peak distress early in the second year reveals an interesting insight into the program. During the first year, students are "learning how to learn" in the PCC environment, as well as preparing for the IB experience. During the IB experience, they are frequently exposed to how little they actually understand and how much they need to learn. Thus, on returning to campus, Board anxiety is acute.

"During IB it really became apparent to me how little anatomy I had learned. During that first year, it was easy to convince yourself that you were learning a lot, and to avoid dealing with the subjects

*you didn't like. But when you come back to school and have Boards
facing you . . . it makes you very anxious."*

Students' initial views toward their curricula were modified by
their particular track. Students in the conventional curriculum believed
more in the need to learn the facts to apply them later on, while students
in PCC believed in applying the basic sciences from early in their
medical education. Consistent differences showed up in the students'
attitudes toward the relevance of their education to their future careers.
Students in PCC placed greater value on, and saw more relevance in,
their educational experiences than did the students in the conventional
curriculum.

Although there are attempts at socialization between the two
groups, contact is, for the most part, minimal in the first two years.
There are simply too few shared experiences. When students do come
together formally, as in the periodic, brief, behavioral science courses,
their stereotypes of one another are often confirmed rather than dis-
credited. For example, after one such course, conventional-track students complained that PCC students asked too many questions and often
disrupted the flow of the lectures. PCC students, on the other hand, felt
that the lectures were intolerable:

> *"It was really uncomfortable after a while. I found myself slipping
> back into an old pattern of sitting in lectures and letting them tell me
> what I need to know. I was bored. I found myself relying on lectures
> even though I knew I could learn the material more efficiently and
> thoroughly by myself."*

Students saw some of the faculty as dichotomizing PCC and
conventional-track students during the first two years. One PCC student
complained:

> *"One faculty member came up to a group of us (PCC students) and
> said, 'Well, the fate of PCC is riding on your shoulders.' I felt as
> though I was struggling just to get through, not also defending the
> entire existence of PCC. It was a little overwhelming."*

Another student recalled:

> *"I was working with one faculty member who was having difficulty
> with PCC, and I felt as though I had to constantly defend the
> program. He saw me as not knowing anything, and would refer to*

> *the conventional curriculum whenever I made a mistake. I felt as*
> *though even if I were perfect he would have told me how much*
> *better I'd be if I had been in the conventional track."*

Conventional-track students have also noted this problem when running up against certain faculty members favoring PCC. One student described an incident which he felt characterized some of the faculty attitudes toward the conventional track:

> *"When I went to talk with Dr. X. because I was having some*
> *problems understanding the material, he kept holding up the PCC*
> *approach as an answer to my problems. 'Now in PCC, students do*
> *this, they do that, they learn this, they learn that.' I felt like*
> *reminding him that I was a conventional-track student. I felt really*
> *uncomfortable because I think he is a really good teacher."*

When students from both tracks come together on third year clerkships, it may be their attitudes rather than their technical skills that distinguish them. While conventional-track students are newly discovering their roles as student physicians and contending with the anxiety and the lack of confidence of their house officers, PCC students' self-image as student doctors has solidified early enough to endure the stresses generated by house staff attitudes. Their experiences in IB leave them with an awareness of the limitations of tertiary care in the broader health care delivery system. They have "special" knowledge of what medicine is really like outside the hospital and medical school. As a result, their attitudes toward the clerkship rotations seem less strained.

Conventional-track students, coming from a much more passive learning environment, rely on house staff for teaching, yet house staff may not be consistent in their willingness or ability to teach. This leaves many conventional-track students quite frustrated.

Conventional-track students frequently characterize PCC students as "brown-nosers" and "too eager to please," while PCC students often characterize conventional-track students as "uptight" and "too competitive." In fact, they come from dissimilar milieus where the rules for student behavior are drastically different. While a low profile may have had survival value for conventional-track students in their preclinical years, it is inappropriate on the wards, where students are rewarded for high interaction and assertiveness. PCC students, on the other hand, have learned to seek a highly interactive learning environment among peers. They are accustomed to being in the spotlight, going to the blackboard to reason through a posed question. For them, many students can learn from one patient problem, as in a tutorial. Yet on the wards, this same sharing attitude can meet with resentment from conventional-track students who perceive the behavior as "horning in" or "showing them up."

Although both student groups evolve in response to certain structural demands and conflicts, both are functional within their own environments. However, when both come together, the differences come into conflict. Over time, as all students gain comfort in their roles as student physicians and gain more comfort being in an active learning environment, the groups tend to meld.

Faculty Attitudes toward PCC

Few medical school faculty have ever received special preparation for teaching (Cantrell, 1973; Jason & Westberg, 1982). The advent of PCC and its need to enlist the participation of many faculty across a variety of disciplines, in a new curricular method, focused considerable faculty attention on educational options.

PCC's request of faculty for teaching service prodded faculty to take a stand on their beliefs. Some were instant converts to the new methods, some took a wait-and-see attitude, and others were, and have remained, adamantly opposed to the program. The longitudinal study surveyed the attitudes of basic and clinical science faculty recruited to tutor in the program. This role provides a faculty member with the fullest exposure to PCC's educational methods, and also requires the greatest personal responsibility for student learning. However, a faculty member accustomed to, and successful in, traditional, didactic teaching, must undergo a substantial role adjustment when now asked to facilitate a student-centered learning group.

Twenty faculty members (ten basic scientists and ten clinicians), who, over a two-year period, taught in the conventional track and who also tutored in the experimental track, were asked to compare tracks in terms of strengths and weaknesses vis-à-vis student performance and educational methods. Chi square was used to test whether there were significant differences between: (1) basic and clinical scientists on their attitudes toward the two tracks, and (2) tutors' perceptions of PCC and the conventional track teaching and evaluation methods. No differences were found between clinical and basic scientists on their observation of the two tracks. As a group, however, they found that conventional-track methods were significantly better able to evaluate students' scientific knowledge ($x^2_4 = 8.94$, $4df$, $p < .05$), but that PCC methods were significantly better able to evaluate students' problem-solving ability ($x^2_4 = 26.08$, $4df$, $p < .001$) and self-motivated learning ($x^2_4 = 27.46$, *df*, $p < .001$). The faculty overwhelmingly (95 percent) desired to tutor again.

This questionnaire was given very early in PCC's development, when most faculty had had little prior contact with the program. These early participants became involved in PCC out of curiosity and a desire to learn a different methodology of teaching. Later recruits, however, may have become involved for different reasons, necessitating a continued study of faculty attitudes toward PCC.

After an experimental pediatric ward rotation on which the entire PCC class of 1983 rotated together, the Pediatric Department faculty were asked to compare the performance of students educated in the problem-based curriculum with that of conventionally prepared students. In addition to the traditional evaluation form, a post-clerkship questionnaire was developed and administered to all Pediatric faculty, asking them to compare the PCC students with the conventional-track students on nine items: (1) basic science knowledge, (2) application of the basic science information to clinical problems, (3) ability to review current research, (4) clinical skills, (5) ability to work with a team, (6) ability to work with peers, (7) enthusiasm for learning, (8) ability to work independently, and (9) level of maturity. The post-clerkship questionnaire was completed by 86 percent of the faculty. They rated performance of the PCC students significantly higher than that of their conventional-track peers on each of the nine items (Figure 10.5). Sample pediatric faculty comments about the PCC students are as follows:

> *"With our regular track, when faculty meet with their two assigned students, all the interest and work comes from the faculty, and it gets very boring. With our [problem-based] students, they run things, and it gets the faculty turned on."*

> *"These students are able to assume more independent responsibility for their own learning, they can integrate their knowledge better . . . they use the library and other resources better."*

> *"I've taken away a great deal from my contact with them and use it in other settings. I'm now more honest in evaluating regular-track students and Pediatric residents. I now ask for their opinions and their reasoning when a question is asked, before I jump in and tell them what to do. I find I'm learning more from and about my students and residents this way and it's more stimulating."*

The enthusiasm among the Pediatrics faculty was tempered by the chairman, who cautioned against making overgeneralizations about the experience. He felt the degree of student and faculty enthusiasm could

Figure 10.5. Rate of performance by 18 pediatric faculty of conventional- vs. problem-based-track students rotating on third-year Pediatric clerkship.

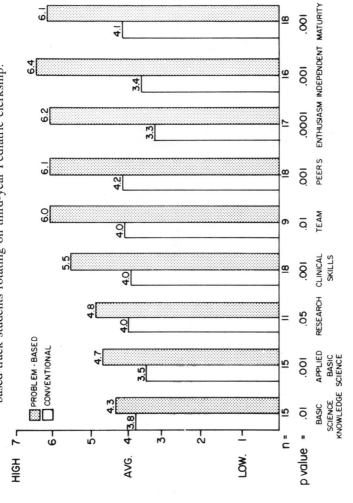

have been as much a result of all the PCC students once again working together as a group as it was a result of their desire to learn.

Many faculty who have not participated in PCC as tutors are less sanguine about the program. While most find some value in the idea of PCC as an educational experiment, there are themes that recur in their criticisms:

1. The heavy teaching burden placed upon participating faculty who must now teach in both tracks interferes with time for their research and perhaps later promotion.
2. Student evaluation in PCC is "soft" and "impressionistic," and it becomes exceedingly difficult to identify strengths and deficiencies in a student's knowledge base.
3. Because the PCC curriculum is student-centered, there is no assurance that students will progress without great gaps in their medical knowledge.
4. PCC students spend too much time learning on their own and not enough time consulting with faculty members who are expert in the students' areas of study.
5. Student-centered learning is not for every student, only for particularly mature, motivated, and scientifically knowledgeable ones.
6. This kind of learning threatens the value and perhaps the very existence of basic science departments, since the departments are without a formal teaching role, serving only as occasional consultants to the students.
7. Early, positive results and enthusiasm on the part of participating students and faculty are better attributed to the Hawthorne effect (positive influence of any change, and of the experimenter's interest in it) than to the educational principles and methods used by PCC.

Sample criticisms of PCC are reflected in the following quotes concerning student–faculty relationships, evaluation methods, and degree of students' responsibility for learning. Some faculty felt that PCC students were treated specially, and were, more often than not, overprotected through the first two years of school.

> *"The PCC students are being treated like a privileged class of students. They are in almost daily contact on a personal basis with a faculty member. They socialize with PCC faculty and many are on a first-name basis. (Wouldn't it be nice if every student could do*

this?) The student–faculty ratio in the PCC program is high. PCC students have their first choices in their selection of electives . . . The point I am emphasizing is that the PCC students belong to a privileged class. They are getting champagne on a beer budget."

Perhaps the most frequently expressed comment among faculty centered on techniques of student assessment. Because assessment in PCC appeared to them so subjective, emphasizing process rather than content, faculty expressed concern about its validity:

"I propose that a 'content'-oriented format be included in the Individual Process Assessment (IPA) [a two-day evaluation administered every two months (see Chapter 8)]. This additional examination should account for at least 15 percent of the overall Year I grades. I propose that at least three basic scientists meet with a tutorial group and quiz/exam the students on the basic science issues relevant to the IPA. If we accept this format, we will have some expert evaluators for the basic science issues relevant to the IPA. These experts will be able to evaluate process as well as content."

But for faculty, perhaps, the most salient issue was one of control:

"I think PCC is a good alternative, but only an alternative. I am not one of the evangelists. One of the main problems is that faculty have no control over the teaching methodology or over the content being taught or the manner in which students are assessed."

Faculty attitudes toward the two tracks needs to be further assessed to determine whether attitudes change over time. For example, does faculty exposure to PCC change their attitude toward students as well as toward the manner in which they teach and evaluate? Although there is currently a substantial move toward incorporating PCC methods into the conventional curriculum, the question remains whether the attitudes and values of PCC will accompany the methods in such a change.

What We Have Learned

1. *The need for independence of the program evaluators.* Although a productive relationship needs to be established between program evaluators and program planners, an independent role for the evaluation team must be clearly defined and supported. This is a particularly difficult task when it is

the planners of the experiment who are funding the evaluation team. Further, program planners may feel pressured to broadcast favorable results prematurely before data collection or analysis is complete. The study subjects' perception of evaluators' independence and objectivity is especially important to the subjects of a study.

2. *The problem of evaluation legitimacy.* Because the evaluation has been financially supported by PCC, it was perceived by many as biased and a part of the experiment itself, rather than as an evaluation of medical education within the School of Medicine. The program evaluation thus had to deal with its own issues of legitimacy. This made it difficult to develop an adequate comparative research design, for conventional-track students were not easily accessible for study.

3. *The complicating variable of student self-selection in a study design.* The program evaluation team was struck by the power of self-selection of students into their preferred track as a factor influencing study results. The team had simply not taken into account a sufficient number of variables in selecting its matched group in the conventional track. This left much of the original data suspect but later led to a cleaner study design in which all acceptable applicants to PCC would be randomized into each track. The ideal experimental design—randomization of all admitted medical students into either a control or experimental group—was ethically and legally impossible.

4. *The need for institutional support for program evaluation.* Typical of all longitudinal research, the program was bedeviled from its outset by an inability to ensure that all students in the study would complete the test instruments on a preassigned schedule. While the more flexible PCC schedule permitted fairly good compliance with program evaluation needs, little time was freed up in the conventional track for this purpose. The medical school as a whole simply had not assumed ownership over longitudinal evaluation.

Experience at Other Schools

McMaster, the first major problem-based medical school, channeled its energy into program development, with less attention paid to comprehensive program assessment. Thus, McMaster describes itself as an innovation rather than an experiment. Much of their program evaluation research uses retrospective evaluation techniques.

The school recently assessed medical graduates' perceptions of how well their medical curriculum prepared them for postgraduate training (Woodward & Ferrier, 1983). Graduates felt very well prepared, compared to fellow postgraduate trainees, in the areas of independent learning, self-evaluation, problem-solving skills, and competence in dealing with social and emotional needs of patients. These are key goals for the McMaster curriculum. However, the graduates felt relatively weak in general basic science content areas, especially in the areas of pharmacology and therapeutics.

The program attempted to assess McMaster medical school graduates by soliciting the judgments of their immediate clinical supervisors (Woodward & McAuley, 1981; Woodward & Ferrier, 1983). Data were collected on 48 graduates of one class. Toward the end of the internship year, a comparison was made between the graduates' self-assessments of their overall preparation for internship compared to their fellow trainees, and supervisors' global assessments of their performance compared with their fellow interns. While there was little agreement between McMaster graduates, in general, graduates' positive self-assessments of their preparation were confirmed by their supervisors.

Elements in Michigan State University's problem-based Track II program evaluation have paralleled many of those in PCC, but a unique and vital component of their evaluation capability was the well-institutionalized Office of Medical Education Research and Development (OMERAD), a national leader in this arena (Jason & Westberg, 1982). As in the New Mexico group, MSU's evaluators had the opportunity to compare students in different educational tracks: Track I (conventional) and Track II (problem-based). However, students were self-selected and no attempt was made to assign matching groups within the tracks.

Over the past ten years, 35 percent of first-year students have selected Track II, with two exceptions—19 percent the first year, 53 percent the last. Curiously, this range is comparable to the percentages of admitted students in New Mexico who select PCC. Like PCC, Track II tends to attract more women than Track I (39 percent versus 33 percent at MSU, 41 percent versus 33 percent at UNM). Important reasons for selecting Track II were educational learning style and flexible time. The strongest influence on decision-making was the opinions of upper classmen. The next strongest influence was personal experience with both modes of learning in the introductory phase.

There is no comparative assessment of cognitive performance between students in each track during the first two years because, as in New Mexico, the tracks are totally separated after the introductory phase, and students do not take common examinations. Thus, the first possible comparison is National Boards—Part I, which became mandatory in 1980. This is now taken by all students at the end of the second year. Overall performance, as in New Mexico, shows no significant difference between tracks. But in contradistinction to New Mexico, the Track II students have significantly higher subsection scores in physiology, biochemistry, and behavioral science than Track I students. Jones et al. theorized that the higher behavioral science scores reflect the heavier emphasis on this subject within the curriculum. Higher physiology and biochemistry scores reflect the fact that Track I students take these subjects early in the first year and see little of that subject matter thereafter, whereas for Track II students biochemistry and physiology are woven through focal problems throughout the two years (Jones et al., 1983).

In a pass/fail grading system, there was little means to compare students on their clinical performance. There was a suggestion that Track II students did better. An indirect measure is the number who have failed the clinical phase—eight from Track I, one from Track II. However, results of content examinations based at the end of each clerkship showed no significant difference. There has been no systematic assessment of the noncontent components of clerkship evaluation. In surveying residency directors about the performance of first-year residents from either track, again, no significant differences emerged.

Finally, career choice of students graduating from the two tracks shows that a higher percentage of students completing Track II entered family practice, pediatrics, and psychiatry, whereas a higher percentage of students in Track I entered surgery.

Implications

There is a need for careful, longitudinal evaluation of problem-based learning programs. While emphasis and funding to date have focused on program implementation, a thrust toward innovation must now be matched by energy devoted to evaluation.

Numerous variables affect problem-based learning programs, such as past experience and self-selection of the program by students, climate for faculty teaching, and level of institutional support. Thus evaluators cannot limit their assessment to student performance or attitudes. Such programs must be analyzed broadly in terms of multiple student and faculty variables, prevailing political and economic forces, and how closely results match program goals.

Because virtually all innovations must respond pragmatically to their environment, it is difficult to maintain a fixed, original study design. Results are very difficult to interpret. It is important for the evaluation design to build flexibility and creativity into the assessment of such a dynamic system. There is thus need to document change (qualitative) as well as simply recording test results (quantitative).

From program outset an attempt should be made to identify a control group of students to strengthen interpretation of the study. And the threat to the independence and objectivity of the evaluation team from program pressure to report favorable results must be resisted.

References

Cantrell, J. (1973). How do medical staff learn to teach? *Lancet, 2,* 734.

Howell, R. E. (1979). Evaluation for dissemination: the rural leadership development project. In J. Lindquist (Ed.), *Increasing the impact of social innovations funded by grant making institutions.* Battle Creek: W. K. Kellog Foundation.

Jason, H., & Westberg, J. (1982). *Teachers and teaching in U.S. medical schools.* East Norwalk, Conn.: Appleton-Century-Crofts.

Jones, J. W., Bieber, L. L., Echt, R., Scheifley, V., & Ways, P. O. (1983). *A problem-based curriculum—10 years experience.* Paper presented at the Annual Workshop on Problem-Based Learning, Maastricht, The Netherlands.

Kellner, R., & Sheffield, B. (1973). A self-rating scale of distress. *Psychology Medicine, 3* (1), 88.

Kolb, D. (1976). *Learning style inventory technical manual.* Boston: McBee and Co.

McCaully, M. (1977). *The Myers-Briggs Longitudinal Medical Study: Application of the Myers-Briggs Type Indicator to medicine and other health professions: Monograph II.* St. Chaumberg, Ill.: American Medical Student Associate Foundation.

O'Donnell, M. J. (1982, Nov.). NBME Part I; Possible explanation for performance based on personality type. *Journal of Medical Education, 57,* 868–870.

Otis, G. D., & Weiss, J. K. (1972). *Explorations in medical career choice.* Limited circulation monographic, longitudinal study. Albuquerque: University of New Mexico School of Medicine.

Otis, G. D., & Weiss, J. K. (1973). Pattern of medicine career preference. *Journal of Medical Education, 48,* 1116–1123.

Rezler, A. G. (1974). Attitude changes during medical school: A review of the literature. *Journal of Medical Education, 49,* 1023.

West, M., Mennin, S. P., Kaufman, A., & Faley, W. (1982) Medical students' attitudes toward basic sciences: Influence of a primary care curriculum. *Medical Education, 16,* 188–191.

Woodward, C. A., & Ferrier, B. M. (1983). The content of the medical curriculum at McMaster University, graduate's evaluation of their preparation for postgraduate training. *Medical Education, 17,* 54–60.

Woodward, C. A., & McAuley, R. G. (1981). Final report: Career choices and development of McMaster medical graduates. Grant D. M. 321. Toronto, Ontario: Ontario Ministry of Health.

Woodward, C., & Neufeld, V. (1979). A long range evaluation of curriculum innovation. In A. Hunt & L. Weeks (Eds.), *Medical education since 1960* (pp. 278–299). East Lansing: Michigan State University Foundation.

CHAPTER 11

Cost of Problem-Based Learning

STEWART P. MENNIN AND
NANCY MARTINEZ-BURROLA

"Look, Stew, why don't we just take the best of both tracks and make a hybrid out of them?" I knew what was coming next as the professor, who had spent little time working in PCC, pursued his point. "You guys work your hearts out for the program and you've generated some good ideas, but it would just take too much faculty time to run small-group learning for the whole medical school class."

He went on to propose molding some of the concepts of PCC with the presumed time efficiency of the conventional track. But I wondered—was small-group, problem-based learning really so expensive? How much comparative time and effort were actually spent teaching in each of the tracks? I decided to find out.

Goals

1. To compare the costs of operating a problem-based versus conventional curriculum.
2. To examine financial and institutional benefits of a problem-based versus conventional curriculum.

Introduction

It is widely assumed that small-group, problem-based learning is more expensive and consumes more faculty time than conventional medical education. However, there have been few data to support or refute that assumption.

Innovative educational proposals are evaluated by both universities and government to determine whether the overall benefits will be worth the overall costs. In the current era of shrinking budgets, decisions about educational innovation may be made more on the basis of financial than pedagogical considerations. Thus, it is essential to understand the factors that contribute to the financial costs of medical education.

In the medical school, faculty salaries comprise a lion's share of educational costs. In addition, the cost of other factors which are essential to medical education, such as research and patient-related activities, must be included.

There have been several attempts to measure the costs of medical education (Carrol, 1958; Hilles, 1973; Stoddart, 1973), but each study has been hampered by the necessity of teasing apart the educational portions of activities such as ward rounds, which may contain some elements of education, patient care, and research. These methodological problems were minimized at New Mexico, because the measurements were made for only the first, nonclinical year. Thus an account needed to be made of the hours devoted to teaching efforts. The comparison of faculty time devoted to each of the two tracks, PCC and conventional, would be indicative of the relative cost of each track. The task was to document the faculty time devoted to each of the two curricula during the first year of medical school.

Methods of Collecting Data:
Conventional Track

Since the combined coursework of the Anatomy, Biochemistry, and Physiology Departments represents 91 percent of the coursework in the first year in the conventional track, a detailed record of the teaching efforts of the full-time faculty in each of these departments was developed. Only the efforts that related to actual instruction of medical students were documented. An interview was conducted with each faculty member who had teaching responsibilities in each of the three departments. These 22 faculty members detailed the time they spent in each of two categories of instruction-related activity—contact time and preparation time.

Contact time refers to the time in which faculty are in actual contact with the students and consists of scheduled class time, such as lectures (including attending other faculty lectures), laboratories, and quizzes and nonscheduled time such as office interviews and extra time spent in laboratories. Preparation time is that time spent preparing for student contact and includes such activities as writing or revising lectures, preparing for laboratory exercises, and writing, revising, or grading examinations (Table 11.1).

Methods of Collecting Data:
Problem-Based Curriculum

There is a broad range of educational roles for faculty in the problem-based curriculum. These include tutoring, evaluating, circuit riding to rural preceptorship sites, acting as a faculty resource, serving as a discipline representative, and participating in special sessions, such as Clinical Skills. An activities checklist was developed in which faculty who had contributed to PCC could categorize their time. In PCC, preparation time represented time involved in training workshops, preparing for tutorials and evaluations, and planning and developing the curriculum. Faculty activities in PCC were subdivided into 10 tasks and 46 subtasks (Table 11.2). Data on faculty effort for the problem-based track were verified by each individual.

Table 11.1. Organization of Teaching Activities in the Conventional Curriculum

Contact Time	Preparation Time
Lecture	Lectures: new/old
Laboratory	Laboratory: new/old
Examinations/ quizzes	Examination and quizzes writing/preparing grading/evaluating
Clinical/ correlates	Reading and grading lab reports and term papers
Attending related lectures and labs	Writing and reviewing syllabi/handout material
Other	Planning time

Table 11.2. Organization of Teaching Activities in the Problem-Based Curriculum

Tasks	Subtasks	Tasks	Subtasks
I. Clinical skills		VI. Evaluator	28. IPA
II. Committees	1. Administration	VII. Faculty development	29. Tutor workshop
	2. Admissions		30. Evaluator workshop
	3. Clinical Skills		31. Observing tutorials
	4. Curriculum		32. Preceptorship workshop
	5. Discipline Rep.		
	6. Evaluation	VIII. Resource faculty	33. Tutorial resource
	7. Evaluation Review		34. Individual resource
	8. Phase IB		
	9. Phase III	IX. Tutor	35. Regular
	10. Policy		36. Co-tutor
	11. Research		37. Substitute
	12. Tutorial		

III. Circuit rider

13. Circuit Ride
14. Site Selection
15. Circuit Rider Meetings

IV. Curriculum development

16. Case Selection
17. Issues Development
18. Simulated Patient
19. Community Medicine Week

V. Discipline problem sessions

20. Anatomy
21. Behavioral science
22. Biochemistry
23. Microbiology
24. Pathology
25. Pharmacology
26. Physiology
27. Radiology

X. Public relations

38. Conference
39. Presentation
40. Publication
41. Visitors
42. Workshop facilitator
43. Workshop attendance
44. Visiting other schools
45. Grants
46. Other

Results

The study was made of the first year of both tracks during the 1983–1984 academic year. During that year there were 20 students in the first year of PCC and 53 students in the first year of the conventional track.

During the first year of the conventional track, students are in class for 40.4 weeks, while during the first year for PCC student activities require 44.0 weeks. The students in both tracks spend their first two weeks together in a course combining Emergency Medicine, Biometry, and Interviewing. At the conclusion of this course, students enter the conventional or PCC track. The total hours documented in the conventional track represent 91 percent or 34.9 weeks of the remaining actual class time. The curricular comparison was therefore calculated for 34.9 weeks for the conventional track and 42 weeks for PCC. For the purposes of discussion, each of these later durations is referred to as a curriculum year.

The comparison was made using a variation of the approach described in the National Academy of Sciences study (Institute of Medicine, 1974). Data were expressed in terms of faculty hours per curriculum week per student. We feel that these results best represent and enable a comparative cost of the two tracks.

For the conventional track, it was found that 22 faculty spent a total of 6,603 hours in teaching and teaching-related activities during the curriculum year. There was considerable variation in the amount of time devoted to education between the departments as well as between faculty in each department (Table 11.3). The faculty hours per curric-

Table 11.3.   Teaching Time during the First Year: Conventional Curriculum

Department	No. of Faculty	Total Hours[a]	Mean % Annual Time Per Faculty Member in Each Department
Anatomy	9	3236	18.7
Biochemistry	5	1627	15.6
Physiology	8	1740	11.2
TOTAL	22	6603	15.2 ± 1.2[b]

[a]Contact time plus preparation time.
[b]Average percent effort of all 22 faculty $\pm$ S.E.M.

ulum week per student was therefore 6,603 hours divided by 34.9 weeks divided by 53 students = 3.57 hours/week/student.

For PCC, the calculation was a little more complex. The first year is divided into Phase IA, which lasts 26 weeks of the curriculum year, and Phase IB, which lasts the remaining 16 weeks. Phase IA is spent on campus, but Phase IB is spent at community-based preceptor sites.

The 26 weeks of Phase IA require the expenditure of 2,144 hours of faculty time. Therefore, the expenditure per week per student was 2,144 hours/26 weeks/20 students = 4.12 hours/week/student. Note that in Phase IA, PCC required 15 percent *more* hours per week per student than did the conventional track, for which the amount was 3.57 hours/week/student. The size of this difference reflects the fact that Phase IA is the most faculty-intensive segment of PCC.

During Phase IB the students are off campus at preceptorship sites. The preceptors are not paid, and thus their time is not included in the expenditure calculations. Faculty time is still expended, however, in activities such as circuit riding, site selection, curriculum development, and telephone consultation. The expenditure of faculty time was 942 hours for Phase IB. The expenditure per week per student was therefore 942 hours/16 weeks/20 students = 2.94 hours/week/student.

Combining the expenditures for Phase IA and IB, the amounts are as follows: Total faculty hours = 2,144 + 942 = 3,086 hours. Total weeks = 26 + 16 = 42 weeks. Expenditure per week per student was therefore, 3,086 hours/42 weeks/20 students = 3.67 hours/week/ student. This is only 3 percent greater than the comparable amount of 3.57 hours/week/student in the conventional track (Figure 11.1).

Preparation versus Contact Time

What emerged from this study was that in our faculty-centered, subject-oriented conventional curriculum an average of 61 percent of the total time devoted to teaching-related activities took place in the *absence* of students. Figure 11.2 illustrates the amount of contact and preparation time which occurred in the three departments studied. Overall, only 39 percent of the total hours were recorded as contact hours. In contrast, in PCC, 72 percent of the total time devoted by faculty to education was spent *with* the students. In a problem-based, student-centered curriculum, tutoring is the most time-consuming activity (Figure 11.3). This high ratio of student contact time to total education time is also typical of other PCC activities. For example, approximately 80 percent of faculty total time devoted to evaluation and to special problem sessions was spent with students.

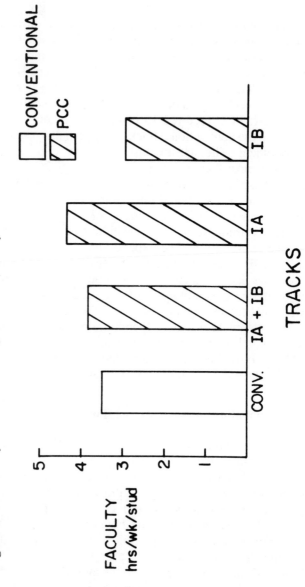

Figure 11.1. Faculty hours/week/student: first curriculum year.

Figure 11.2. Distribution and breakdown of teaching time in the first year of conventional track.

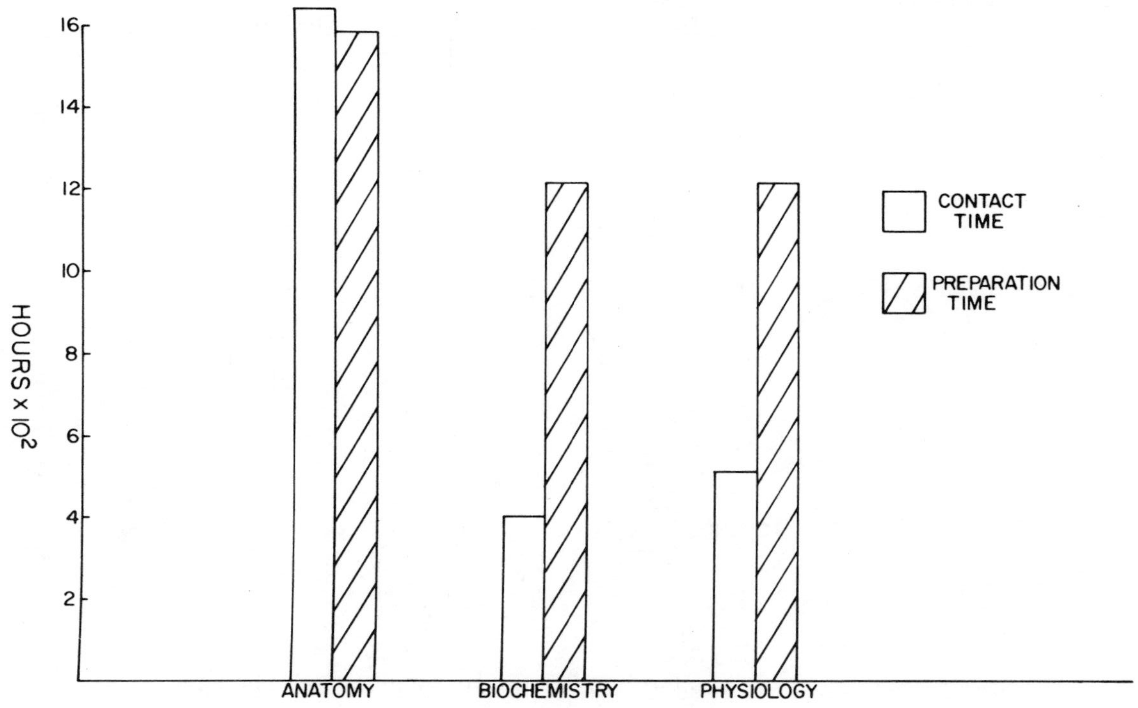

CONTACT TIME

PREPARATION TIME

PHYSIOLOGY

BIOCHEMISTRY

ANATOMY

HOURS x 10²

16
14
12
10
8
6
4
2

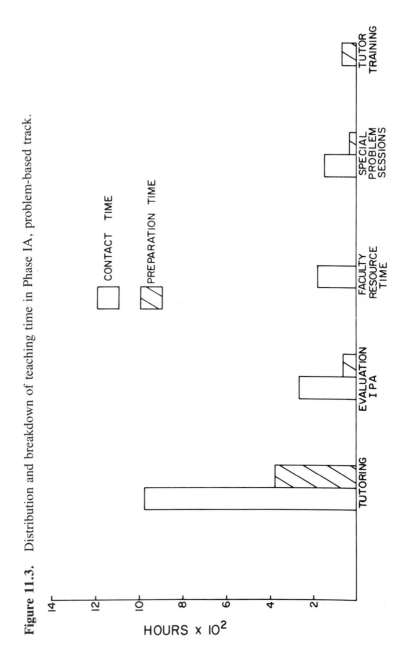

Figure 11.3. Distribution and breakdown of teaching time in Phase IA, problem-based track.

Future Study Plans

What are our plans for the immediate future of this study? Teaching efforts of both curricula in the second year will be documented. There are important differences in the second year: (1) In the second year of PCC, most tutorials meet twice instead of three times a week. On the other hand, students spend eight more weeks at the medical center than they did in the first year. (2) In the second year of the conventional track, the fall semester is taught primarily by basic science faculty (65 percent), while in the spring 79 percent of the teaching is done by clinicians. It is notable that the percentage of basic and clinical science to clinical faculty in the second year of the problem-based track is similar to that of the conventional track (Table 11.4).

The tutorial group ratio of one faculty member to five students is not inviolate. If, for example, the tutorial group were enlarged to six or seven students per tutor, as in many other problem-based programs, the cost of the program would be substantially reduced.

Benefits

Up until now we have considered only the costs of problem-based and conventional track education. What about their benefits?

Conventional Track

The conventional track is a time-honored approach to education with which many faculty and students are comfortable. They know how to function within it and what to expect. Their roles are clearly defined, and

Table 11.4. Percentage of Basic[a] and Clinical Science Faculty Teaching during the First Two Years of Medical School

		Basic Scientists	Clinical Scientists
Year 1	Conventional track	73	27
	Problem-based track[b]	68	32
Year 2	Conventional track	38	62
	Problem-based track	31	69

[a]Pathology is included as a basic science department.
[b]PCC time is tutorial time.

the road to "success" is plainly marked. Satisfaction and comfort with a well-defined system of education is a definite plus. The lecture mode of transmitting an organized body of information is, in the hands of an expert, highly efficient. It can serve to inspire and challenge the listener. In addition, lecture and faculty-centered education can serve to assure the faculty that no major gaps exist in the information to which students have been exposed. The evaluation system clearly states what is necessary in order to achieve a satisfactory performance. Faculty and administrators can point to the class schedule as written documentation of their teaching contribution.

As a rule, teaching in the conventional track generates little income. However, there have been exceptions. For example, research dollars in educational development have been awarded for a genetics learning system and a microbial genetics learning series, both self-teaching, slide–tape programs, developed by Dr. Tom Baker, Department of Microbiology, with the aid of funds from the National Fund for Medical Education and National Science Foundation. Other funded projects have included Pulmonary Training, Transfusion Medicine Education, and Cancer Education grants.

Problem-Based Track

The problem-based track has resulted in a wide spectrum of benefits beyond the training of physicians for the State of New Mexico. It has enriched the educational environment of the university by stimulating change toward problem-based learning in the conventional track. The presence of parallel curricular tracks has created a laboratory in which to study medical education, examine curricular innovations and evaluate variations of the learning process.

The problem-based track has become a well-spring for faculty development. Workshops for training tutors have provided faculty with skills in new teaching and evaluation methodologies. Tutoring in small groups has offered many faculty valuable insight into alternative teaching options. All of these activities have served to introduce faculty to the problem-based approach to education (Table 11.5). This training has all been built into the program's operating budget and did not require a separate expense. Several faculty members have chosen to remain at UNM in spite of offers of employment at other universities. They claim that a key factor in their decision to remain has been the personal satisfaction and enjoyment obtained through the problem-based curriculum.

The problem-based curriculum developed new linkages and broadened those that already exist between community health care

Table 11.5. Faculty Participation in PCC

	1979/80	*1980/81*	*1981/82*	*1982/83*
Administrative faculty (Policy Committee)	8	14	18	12
Tutors[a]				
Basic science	3	8	9	8
Clinical science	5	10	18	19
Other[b]			1	2
Evaluators				
Basic science	11	15	22	17
Clinical	15	15	16	28
Other[c]				6
TOTAL	42	62	84	92

[a]Includes co-tutors.
[b]Other includes School of Medicine faculty with Ph.D.s in areas other than the basic sciences and faculty from other schools.
[c]Other includes those listed in footnote b above plus UNM/SOM Residents.

providers, the state, and the School of Medicine. It has helped the School of Medicine gain national and international recognition for efforts in education. As private funding has declined, the school, via state legislative appropriations, has assumed support of program costs— an important measure of institutional acceptance of the experimental track. PCC has also generated grant support and stimulated multiple research projects related to education and health care delivery (Table 11.6).

Small-group, problem-based learning is now a regular part of conventional-track courses in pathology, endocrinology, behavioral sciences, and physiology. A variety of well-trained simulated patients have been developed in PCC. A steadily increasing demand for them is occurring in the departments of Internal Medicine, Psychiatry, Surgery and Family Medicine. They are used in both training and evaluation of residents. Evaluation forms developed in PCC are used for all third- and fourth-year students (Table 11.7).

Increased access to medical center facilities and the medical center library for preceptors has helped to forge a stronger relationship between the school and the outlying communities. Students have gained an increased awareness of the health care needs of the state. One benefit is

Table 11.6. PCC's Record in Attracting Funds to the UNM School of Medicine

A. *PCC Grant Awards*

Kellogg Planning Grant, 1976–78	$ 48,414
First Kellogg, 1978–81	681,034
Second Kellogg, 1981–85	743,659
FIPSE, 1980–83	271,535
Kellogg Documentary Film, 1984–85	49,550
Kellogg, Evaluation, 1984–87	271,800
National Fund for Medical Education, 1982–84	41,830
Total	$2,107,822

B. *PCC Grant Applications (Pending)*

PCC-UNAM Linkage	$ 230,000
FIPSE Dissemination	7,959
WKK Dissemination	40,000
Total	$277,959

C. *PCC-Related Grant Awards*

National Library of Medicine, Information Searching Guides 1981–83	$ 95,133
National Fund for Medical Education, 1982–84	41,830
Total	$136,963

D. *PCC-Related Grant Applications (Pending)*

FIPSE Medical Self-Assessment Center	$ 326,055
Area Health Education Center for N.M.	1,498,923
Kellogg, Community-Based Health Improvement	4,375,982
Total	$6,200,960

Table 11.7. Influence of PCC on Conventional Track

---

1. *Courses in which problem-based learning is now used*
   Introduction to Pathology
   Endocrine II Bloc
   Behavioral Sciences
   Renal II Bloc
2. *PCC's Simulated Patient Program—which departments now use them*
   Internal Medicine (Clinical Science)
   Psychiatry (Behavioral Science Bloc)
   Surgery
   Family Medicine (Resident Evaluation)
3. *Evaluation:* All clinical clerks are now evaluated using forms developed by PCC to include assessment of clinical reasoning.

---

that because of the enjoyment and education that preceptors experience as a result of their interaction with PCC students, the number of preceptors participating in PCC has grown steadily over the past five years.

What If . . . ?

What would happen to costs if the 53 students in the conventional track were to change to a problem-based, student-centered curriculum? Although we would need more tutors, these would come from the faculty pool switching their curricular activities from the conventional track. The real bottleneck in such a changeover would come in Phase IB. It would take considerable time to place an additional 53 students in adequate preceptorship sites for four months around the state of New Mexico. One possible solution to this dilemma would be alternative preceptorships, either in urban clinics or in university research laboratories.

Summary

Careful analysis of the amount of time required to operate each of the curricula during the first year showed that a significant amount of the total teaching time is devoted to preparation for student contact in the conventional track. The opposite is true in the problem-based track, in which 70 to 80 percent of the total faculty time devoted to tutoring, evaluation, special sessions, and resource activities is spent in the presence of the students. When faculty hours per curricular week per student are examined, the problem-based track required virtually the same total time. Based on data obtained during the first part of this continuing study, it is fair to conclude that at the University of New Mexico School of Medicine, the difference between the tracks should be explained on the basis of their educational merits rather than on temporal and financial considerations.

Implications

What we have seen is that contrary to popular assumptions, faculty time devoted to problem-based education is no greater than that devoted to conventional education. In fact, it might prove more attractive to the institution due to the increased faculty–student contact time it fosters and the grants in research it attracts.

Portions of this study have appeared in abstract form, *Proceedings of the 23rd Annual Conference, RIME* (1984, pp. 33–38).

References

Carroll, A. J. (1958). *A study of medical college costs.* Washington, D.C.: Association of American Medical Colleges.

Hilles, W. C. (1973). Program cost allocation and the validation of faculty activity involvement. *Journal of Medical Education, 48,* 805–813.

Institute of Medicine (1974, Jan.). *Report of a Study, Costs of Education in the Health Professions.* Parts I and II. U.S. Department of Health, Education and Welfare; Public Health Service; Health Resources Administration, Bureau of Health Resources Development, Bethesda, Md., and the National Academy of Sciences, Washington, D.C. DHEW Publication No. (HRA) 74–32.

Stoddart, G. L. (1973). Effort-reporting and cost analysis of medical education. *Journal of Medical Education, 48,* 814–823.

CHAPTER 12

International Perspectives

MARTIN P. KANTROWITZ AND ARTHUR KAUFMAN

Caryn and Evan, two PCC students, surveyed the crowded rows of temporary, jerry-built houses papering the hillside overlooking the polluted haze covering Mexico City below. This was the newest community of the disenfranchized immigrants to the city. Its inhabitants were tolerating social dislocation and urban squalor to escape the certainty of grinding poverty and starvation in the countryside.

The students were guided across a narrow dirt path to a cluster of five dwellings built of corrugated metal and wood slats. This cluster had been assigned to a first-year Mexican medical student from the new, community-oriented track of the National Autonomous University of Mexico. Dr. Lievana, a physician-tutor in the new track, told Caryn and Evan the many responsibilities his first-year students had to the inhabitants of this community— keeping health records (e.g., births, immunizations, contraceptive use), identifying environmental risk factors (e.g., faulty wiring, mud slides, sewage disposal, impotable water), and providing health education (e.g., talks on sanitation, advice on eligibility for health benefits, advocacy of the inhabitants' health care needs to the district health clinic).

Caryn and Evan had taken pride in their community health involvement through PCC, but their program hadn't the scope or vision of that of their counterparts in Mexico. Evan wondered

aloud, "Why couldn't we try something like this in Albuquerque?"
This small question eventually led to the building of a major link
between medical schools on either side of the Mexico—United
States border.

Introduction

Doctors find themselves unaccustomed to assess and evaluate the health
care needs and priorities of their own country and its people. They are
incapable of providing or implementing preventive programs. They are
unprepared to work in the slums of the cities or to manage a rural health
care team. (Bollag et al., 1982, p. 282)

This criticism is, perhaps, most evident within developing countries where the discrepancy between the orientation of medical education and the reality of consumer needs is so grossly apparent (King,
1966). Medical educators worldwide are attempting to reorient medical
education toward community health care needs. The differences they
face are often a matter of scale. For example, maldistribution of physicians by geography and specialty is now a problem widely acknowledged in the United States and has generated numerous educational
innovations to redress the imbalance (Odegaard, 1979). The problem is
very much larger, however, in developing countries; for while two-
thirds of the world's population lives in Africa, Asia, and Latin America, they have among them but one-quarter of the world's physicians
(Wolstendholme, 1971).

It is a sizable undertaking to create a major reorientation of a
medical school curriculum. Economic constraints, political climate,
faculty inertia, and issues of territorial control within the medical
institution all pose formidable barriers. It is noteworthy that a sizable
portion of the medical schools worldwide that are conducting major
experiments either in problem-based learning or in community-oriented
primary care are new schools (e.g., McMaster, Maastricht, Suez,
Saudia Arabia, Xochimilco, Mercer, Beersheba). A new school can
attract faculty who are committed to the new philosophy and is less
fettered by the rigidity of tradition and convention. The vast majority of
medical students in the world, however, are educated in conventional
medical schools where the obstacles to change are far greater.

The successes and failures of the varied approaches of medical
schools worldwide can provide a rich data base of experience from
which others can learn. Vehicles for rapid dissemination of such information are needed. It is thus imperative that international networking
be activated among the many interested medical schools.

Characterizing the
Innovative Schools

There are scores of innovative medical school programs worldwide. A sampling of 40 such schools—20 from developing countries and 20 from technically developed countries—appears in Table 12.1. While the majority of innovative programs in technically developed countries originated in schools already in existence, the majority of programs in developing countries were established as a part of the curriculum in newly created schools. It appears that creating change in traditional schools in developing countries is far more difficult. This is ironic, for the palpable need for such change is even more immediate in developing countries. An educator from an innovative medical school program in Fiji commented,

> The medical profession has been caught up with overspecialization at the expense of universal coverage of health services. Time and time again, developing countries have expended valuable resources in establishing medical schools based on models from highly sophisticated and industrialized countries. Even more unfortunately, occasionally these have been adopted wholesale with scant attention to the appropriateness of such training in relation to the existing health service infrastructure within which the graduates will practice. (Pathik & Goon, 1978, p. 96)

Figure 12.1 suggests that whereas the dominant focus of innovative programs in technically developed countries is problem-based learning, in developing countries there is a stronger emphasis on community-oriented medical education.

The underlying problems and forces promoting changes in medical education in developing and technically developed countries are important to review. They not only point out differences in emphasis but suggest fertile terrain for collaboration and networking between the problem-based and community-oriented medical school programs. Two schools, McMaster in Canada and the Institute for Health Sciences in Manila, Philippines, illustrate differences in motivation and program response in technically developed and developing countries.

McMaster is perhaps the oldest of the problem-based medical schools and the most influential in the dissemination of its innovative ideas throughout the world. In 1965, its first dean, John Evans, began to assemble a group of educators to create the new curriculum. Their criticisms of conventional medical education became the driving force behind the student-centered, tutorial-run, problem-based curriculum that emerged. Among the problems identified were the following:

Table 12.1. A Sample of 40 Problem-Based and/or Community-Oriented Medical School Programs Worldwide

| | | Schools in Technically Developed Countries | | | |
| | | Innovation Occurred | | Orientation | |
	Year Program Estab.	In Exist. School	De Novo	Problem-Based	Commun.
North America					
1. McMaster U. Canada	1969		X	X	
2. U. Minnesota, USA	1971	X			X
3. Sophie Davis— CCNY, USA	1972		X		X
4. Michigan State U., USA	1973	X		X	
5. Upper Peninsula, Michigan State U., USA	1974	X		X	X
6. U. of Arizona, USA	1978	X			X
7. U. of New Mexico, USA	1979	X		X	X
8. U. of Colorado, USA	1981	X		X	
9. Southern Illinois U., USA	1981	X		X	
10. Mercer, Georgia, USA	1982		X	X	X
Europe					
1. Pecs, Hungary	1972	X		X	
2. Kuopio, Finland	1972		X	X	X
3. Maastricht, Holland	1974		X	X	
4. Utrecht, Holland	1976	X		X	
5. Moscow, USSR	1976	X		X	
6. Edinburgh, UK	1978	X		X	
7. Southhampton, UK	1978	X		X	
8. Alicante, Spain	1980		X	X	
9. Belfast, N. Ireland	1981	X		X	
Australia					
1. Newcastle, Australia	1978		X	X	X

| | | Schools in Technically Developing Countries | | | |
| | | Innovation Occurred | | Orientation | |
	Year Program Estab.	In Exist. School	De Novo	Problem-Based	Com-mun.
Latin America					
1. Brasilia, Brazil	1972	X		X	X
2. Mexico City, Mex.	1974	X			X
3. Xochimilco, Mex.	1974		X	X	X
Middle East					
1. Hucettepa, Turkey	1967		X		X
2. Aden, Yemen	1975		X	X	
3. Beersheba, Israel	1975		X		X
4. Riyadh, Saudi Arabia	1977	X			X
5. Basrah, Iraq	1978	X			X
6. Wad Medani, Sudan	1978		X	X	X
7. Ismailia, Egypt	1981		X	X	X
Asia					
1. Bangkok, Thailand (Ramashibah)	1969		X		X
2. Khon Kaen, Thailand	1974		X	X	X
3. Suva, Fiji	1975	X		X	
4. U. Manila, Philippines	1976	X			X
5. Katmandu, Nepal	1978				X
6. Panang, Malaysia	1981		X	X	X
Africa					
1. Yaoundi, Cameroon	1970		X		X
2. Ilorin, Nigeria	1978		X	X	X
3. Free Town, Sierra Leone	1979		X	X	X
4. Kumas, Ghana	1981	X		X	X

Figure 12.1. Nature of innovation in 40 problem-based and/or community-oriented medical schools in developing and technically developed countries.

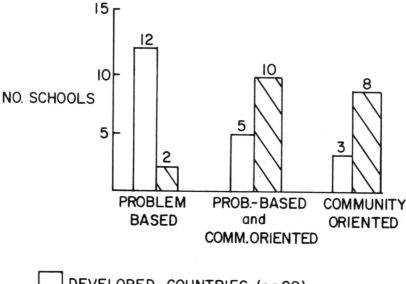

1. A rigid, lock-step curriculum governed by departmental power and influence within the dean's office.
2. A sharp distinction between preclinical and clinical medical sciences.
3. An imbalance in the exposure of students to health problems seen in a teaching hospital versus those seen by physicians among the general population in the community.
4. A divergence in the goals of the university faculties of medicine versus the teaching hospitals and their staffs.
5. A lack of concern about assessing the effectiveness of diagnostic and treatment procedures and the effectiveness with which health care was delivered.
6. A lack of concern in the education programs with the preparation of physicians to provide sensitive, effective, efficient, primary care in the community. (Mustard et al., 1982)

In response, the planning group developed an administrative matrix whereby the educational programs would be administered by a broadly representative faculty group, rather than by particular departments. A flexible curriculum focused on the study of patient problems, thereby ensuring integration of basic and clinical science study. To transfer more responsibility for learning from teachers to students, students were to meet in small tutorial groups, identify their own learning needs from the problems, and spend considerable time in independent study.

Further, to get a better appreciation of the entire health care system, students were to spend time in various community settings. As a consequence, considerable effort was invested in developing joint programs in health care, teaching, and research among the university hospital and all the community hospitals.

To put teeth into the objectives of the new program, the old faculty reward system also had to be changed. The new promotion policy emphasized first a faculty member's need to demonstrate excellence in education. Then he must demonstrate excellence in either research or health services.

A very different set of circumstances motivated the creators of the Institute of Health Sciences (IHS) program at the University of the Philippines (Bonifacio, 1980). While most medical schools in developing countries have been modeled on those in industrialized countries in the Northern Hemisphere, IHS made a radical departure from this norm. The IHS program was established in 1976 with a primary intent of developing various levels of health manpower by utilizing a career-ladder system. While the immediate target areas are the economically depressed and underserved islands of Samar and Leyte, the ultimate objective is to develop models of health manpower development useful for the Philippines as a whole. The country not only suffers from severe physician maldistribution, but approximately 80 percent of graduates of Philippine medical schools leave the country to practice abroad. The great majority of those who stay remain in the cities.

The program is rooted in the islands' *barangays* (the smallest political units of the country). Candidates for health care careers are nominated by leaders from *barangays* in needy areas, usually remote from cities. The students, in turn, pledge to return to their home communities as health workers.

The student then enters a career-ladder program that combines formal instruction with extended periods of community service on the islands. After the first quarter of formal study, the student works in the community for an academic quarter as a medical auxiliary. He evaluates the health services in his *barangay,* in relation to such matters as family planning, nutrition, and sanitation. During this time, with the assistance of the Institute, the student develops linkages with rural health administrators who help supervise and evaluate his work, thus reinforcing the central role of the community in the program.

At succeeding levels, the curriculum introduces increasingly demanding basic science courses. The successful completion of each level permits more advanced certification and entry into further training for careers with greater responsibility and reward. At each level, the student can leave school and enjoy a useful health career in his or her community. The second level, the Community Health Worker program, for example, incorporates training in midwifery, after which the student is eligible to take the national Midwifery Board Examination.

The third level, Community Health Nursing, takes one year to complete and includes more advanced training in clinical sciences. After completion of the fourth level, the student has achieved the equivalent of a baccalaureate degree. Students who enter the final, three-year phase are in a physician program in which the students shuttle back and forth between the community and the medical school in Manila.

Medical educators worldwide are anxiously awaiting the results of this important experiment in medical education. It is still too early to tell whether the extensive, community-based experiences will motivate the students to return to their underserved island communities. However, there is a general anxiety that the lures of the big city and specialty practice may undermine the purposes of the carefully planned community-based programs.

The Emergence of Networks

The Network of Community-Oriented Educational Institutions for Health Sciences is an international umbrella organization under which many innovative medical school programs, committed to community orientation and problem-based learning, meet and exchange ideas.* It was founded in 1979 at a meeting in Kingston, Jamaica, and has subsequently held meetings in Ballagio, Italy, in 1981 and Havana, Cuba, in 1983. It is currently co-sponsored by the World Health Organization and the Rockefeller Foundation and has almost 50 participating medical schools.

*The address of the Network Central Secretariat is Prof. Dr. J. M. Greep, Dean of the Faculty of Medicine, Rijksuniversiteit Limburg, P.O.B. 616, 6200 MD, Maastricht, The Netherlands.

The Network was established with five main objectives:

1. Strengthening of membership institutions in their realization of community orientation and problem-based learning.
2. Strengthening of individual faculty capacities related to community orientation and problem-based learning.
3. Development of technologies, approaches, methodologies, and tools appropriate to a community-oriented and problem-based educational system.
4. Promoting and coordinating the population-based concepts in the health services system and the educational program.
5. Assisting institutions in countries that have made a political decision to introduce innovations in the training of health personnel.

To these ends, Network members have conducted a series of workshops and conferences on such diverse topics as curriculum development, student evaluation, newer teaching methodologies, and community-based medical education, in such locations as Ismailia in Egypt, Maastricht in the Netherlands, Wad Medani in the Sudan, and Kumas in Ghana.

Network activities can be of critical importance to the development of newer programs. These fledgling programs can profit from the experience of others, and from the stamp of legitimacy from an international organization. In this spirit of interuniversity collaboration, preliminary discussions have developed in the Western Hemisphere between three Network members—the Universidad Autonama Metropolitana–Xochimilco in Mexico, McMaster in Canada, and Universidad del Valle in Columbia. Another link is emerging between schools in the Middle East and Europe involving Ismailia in Egypt, Wad Medani in the Sudan, and Maastricht in the Netherlands.

A Model Network Link

Networking has also played an important role for the Primary Care Curriculum in New Mexico. In 1982, PCC planners learned of an experimental medical school track at the Universidad Nacional Autonoma de Mexico in Mexico City. This is a much larger program than PCC, but it has very similar community-oriented goals. Both programs are attempting to effect institutional change by establishing a separate, community-oriented, medical school track. They both use a tutorial method of instruction. Whereas PCC accepts 20 students per year out of a class of 73, the Mexican program accepts 200 out of a class of approximately 1,500.

The Mexican program, entitled The General Integrated Medical Program (MGI), is decentralized, assigning students in their first two years to four academic units in urban and rural communities adjacent to primary care clinics. Such clinics are selected because of the enormous socioeconomic problems in those communities.

Each tutor supervises the work of 25 students for an entire year. The students work in small groups of five and present their findings to the larger group. Learning is conducted around basic and clinical science modules rather than patient problems, and such study is reinforced and complemented by community service. Over two years, each student is assigned to a cluster of families and to an elementary school. On a weekly basis, the student conducts public health surveys on his assigned families, performs school health screening, and gives health talks to community residents. He identifies illness in the community and brings it to the attention of the clinic. In this fashion, students are able to integrate theory and practice.

In one sample district, each student is assigned to a cluster of flimsy shacks on a hill on the outskirts of the city. These clusters form one of many new communities intended to absorb the burgeoning population of rural poor who migrate to the city for a better life. But most of the inhabitants are without steady work, and they suffer the consequences of social isolation and economic privation. In assessing health risks for this population, students have noted such potential hazards as inadequate immunization levels and improper waste disposal.

This curriculum represents a radical departure from traditional Mexican medical education. It replaces disciplined lectures with modular-based tutorials and places students in a responsible, community-based, caregiving capacity from the beginning of medical school. It emphasizes primary care both by the location of its classrooms (in communities, adjoining primary care clinics) and by the choice of tutors (all primary care physicians).

Preliminary talks between planners of MGI and PCC generated interest in developing contacts between the two programs and their respective institutions. There appeared to be common ground for a closer relationship beyond the similarity in goals and methods of the two programs. The State of New Mexico and the nation of Mexico are, in many respects, natural allies in the quest for medical education aimed at the solution of community health problems. Both share a common border, a comparable climate, and, in part, a common language, history, and ethnic heritage. Both have large, rural, underserved populations.

There has been a series of exchange visits held in Mexico City and Albuquerque. Mutual presentations and observations of each other's programs have taken place. Programmatic and research areas fertile for collaboration have been identified and the Deans of the two medical schools met in Albuquerque and signed a collaborative agreement.

The results of the exchange have been substantial. PCC students have incorporated a modified version of the MGI students' community work by developing a major elementary and secondary school–based health program in Albuquerque in collaboration with the Albuquerque Public School System. In 1984, two MGI faculty spent several weeks working at UNM, and one PCC faculty member spent three months working at UNAM. In 1985, two teams of PCC students, under family practice resident supervision, worked in rural Mexican villages, sharing with their Mexican counterparts skills and approaches to community health problems. MGI faculty are incorporating PCC's clinical skills teaching methodologies into the third and fourth years of their program.

Implications

There is a tide of change in medical education which is of international proportions. Its sources are many—from economic pressures to reduce the cost of care to community pressure to distribute health care resources equitably. It is increasingly apparent that the old models of medical education are simply inadequate to meet the newer expectations regarding the delivery of health care.

Medical education is extremely costly, and the attempts at institutional change require an enormous expenditure of effort with no guarantee of success. The forces opposing change are formidable and are rooted in a system with values that are often quite different from those of the innovators. Thus, it is a timely and necessary development that networks are forming among the innovative schools to share ideas and curriculum and evaluation materials, and to bolster one another's efforts.

References

Bollag, V., Schmidt, H., Fryers, T., & Lawani, J. (1982). Medical education in action: Community-based experience and service in Nigeria. *Medical Education, 16*, 282–289.

Bonifacio, A. F. (1980). University of the Philippines College of Medicine, Philippines: The Institute of Health Sciences, Tacloban. Search for a model. *Public Health Papers, 71* (2), 115–130.

King, M. (1966). *Medical care in developing countries*. New York: Oxford University Press.

Mustard, J. F., Neufeld, V. R., Walsh, W. J., & Cochran, J. (1982). *New Trends in Health Sciences Education, Research and Services: The McMaster Experience*. New York: Praeger.

Odegaard, C. E. (1979). Area health education centers: The pioneering years. *A technical report for the Carnegie Council on Policy Studies in Higher Education*, Berkeley, Calif.

Pathik, B., & Goon, E. (1978). Fiji School of Medicine, Suva, Fiji: From medical assistants to physicians. *Public Health Papers, 70*, 79–96.

Wolstendholme, G. E. (1971). Florence Nightingale—handmaid of civilization. In *Teamwork for World Health*. CIBA Foundation Blueprint. London: J. and A. Churchill.

CHAPTER 13

Institutionalizing Innovation

SAMUEL W. BLOOM

The revision of the formal codes is indeed impressive. Included is a new curriculum, very much in line with current trends toward integration, the introduction of clinical experience earlier in the medical school, and toward elective options. But as I look over the scene as it presents itself today, the nagging question remains: *Are these genuine changes or merely reforms in the classic adaptive mode?* When I am told by one of the department chairmen still on the scene that, as he said, "The same people make the important decisions," my uneasiness is reinforced. Are we seeing . . . a phenomenon that, in my judgment, creates one of the major delusions in the organizational life of our time: *reform without change?* (Bloom, 1973, p. 172)

Kaufman learned this lesson while still a medical student at the Downstate Medical Center[*] in the mid-sixties. His school at that time was the subject of an institutional case study which documented the powerful inertia to change that is inherent in the structure of the modern medical school. Now that he, himself, was challenging the traditional methods and perspectives of medical education, Kaufman recalled the summary warning of the earlier research that unless significant change occurs in the structure of the medical school, the "new bottles of curriculum reform will be filled only with old wine" (Bloom, 1973:173).

[*]State University of New York, Brooklyn, New York.

The Downstate study had been conducted by a sociologist, Samuel W. Bloom. He and Kaufman became friends at Downstate and maintained the friendship throughout the intervening years. It seemed natural, therefore, that Kaufman should consult with his friend about the PCC concept as it was being developed. As early as 1976, Kaufman called (Bloom had moved from Downstate to Mount Sinai School of Medicine in New York) to ask what selection criteria, on the basis of previously published research, would be predictive for the career goals of the initial proposal to Kellogg. Regular informal consultation continued, including a visit to New York by Obenshain, Voorhees, and Kaufman. Finally, in December 1978, the final year of preparation, Bloom was brought to Albuquerque to discuss in detail the plans for evaluation of PCC (then still known as CPC). On that visit, it was agreed that the evaluation ideally should do the following:

1. Monitor the comparative learning of the three comparison groups, using the most appropriate descriptive methods (described above in Chapter 10).
2. Observe, intensively, the full scope of medical school life to identify the operating norms of behavior in all the major subgroups.
3. Feed back for self-study as much information as possible from the evaluation, in short feedback loops for the purpose of directly enhancing and enriching the PCC program itself and making more possible the achievement of its goals. This method is known as "concurrent evaluation" (Moss, 1970).

Convinced that the innovative approach of PCC would have special interest for both the medical profession and the government, it was agreed that it was just as important to document *how* it would work as it was to measure its effects. Such a process analysis would intentionally seek to uncover precisely those problems that participants are likely to be unaware of until they have caused damage. Instead of spending all of its evaluative resources on the study of outcomes, the ongoing observation and description of PCC was designed to fine-tune its organizational development. It was, in other words, intended to help PCC avoid the trap of "old wine in new bottles."

To conduct such an evaluation in full scale, however, is costly. Seen as the "external evaluation," the defined task was to measure and describe the experience of PCC in terms that would allow the field to judge a program that might have replication value to medical education in general. Asked to calculate the cost, Bloom's initial annual budget, using only locally available personnel working with part-time external consultants, was close to $60,000. Considering the scope of the program, this estimate would seem to be a modest cost. However, the available resources were limited, and the choice, much like similar educational innovations such as the McMasters curriculum, was to commit them primarily to the implementation of the educational program rather than to the evaluation. In the end, the study was conducted with less than half the original estimate, but instead of an on-site senior social scientist to supervise the work, Bloom himself became the external consultant. This involved about three week-long visits to Albuquerque annually, plus telephone, correspondence, and visits by PCC personnel to New York. Dr. Maggi West became the full-time field observer and coordinator. Together, West and Bloom gathered the data that are reported here as the story of the institutionalization of PCC.

As George Miller, himself one of the most seasoned veterans of educational research and innovation in American medical schools, recently observed, "Very few schools have managed to establish any effective system for continuously monitoring anything more than the content of instructional programs; and even here the effort has been sporadic and attended by indifferent success" (Miller, 1980:210). That PCC accepted the mandate to chronicle its own detailed history, candidly looking at the face of its failures as well as its triumphs, is demonstrated in the whole of this book. This chapter, therefore, in order not to be redundant, must be selective, more interpretive than descriptive. Tracing the patterns of PCC's development from an experimental to an accepted local program at the University of New Mexico, it will attempt to show with illustrations the major challenges that occurred and to relate them to a model of innovation in higher education.

The Attitude Climate
in the Beginning: 1979–1980

As it moved from planning to implementation, PCC had clarified its goals in two major categories:

1. *The outcomes in professional behavior.* PCC was designed to produce primary care doctors, specially prepared for rural practice, and trained at the highest level of technical competence for the delivery of modern medicine.
2. *The experience of becoming a doctor.* The character of the teaching–learning process was organized to activate the learner, to enhance the significance of the basic sciences by pre-

senting them always in a clinically relevant context, to provide a learning experience that directly simulated the types of
problem-solving demands that would be met in professional
life, and to establish the equal importance of interpersonal
skills and psychosocial factors in medicine.

Concerning the first purpose, as shown earlier in this book, there was
strong pressure, both locally and nationally. Despite the pioneering,
community-oriented perspective of the University of New Mexico
School of Medicine from its very beginning, serious questions were
being raised in the state about whether the medical school was fulfilling
its original purposes to supply more primary care physicians to rural
practices. The data were not encouraging. There was a perceived crisis
of manpower distribution by the State of New Mexico and by the United
States Congress. An attempt to deal with this crisis, therefore, was one
rationale to try PCC.

Less clear were the attitudes toward the second type of objective,
concerned with the experience of *becoming a doctor*. In his early field
visits, Bloom found evidence that PCC had won its right to a trial more
for its educational side-effects than for its central purposes. For example, a number of the school's leading faculty and administrators
embraced PCC essentially because of what they expected would be its
"Hawthorne effect." More precisely, they meant that the conditions of
an educational experiment would energize and add enthusiasm to medical education at New Mexico. "It is worth it to have a program that
excites the faculty." "Enthusiasm is important for teaching." Such were
the typical comments.

There was also evidence that the medical students who were
recruited to the University of New Mexico were seen by its faculty as
themselves the cause of basic educational problems. Instead of PCC
being seen as an exciting method of capturing the enthusiasm of students
who are basically able but discouraged by the didacticism of the existing
curriculum, it was seen more as a way to excite the faculty toward a
greater effort with "reluctant" (and by implication, not so capable)
students. The opposite side of this same attitude was the question raised
as to whether medical students, "especially the New Mexico student,"
are "properly prepared for the PCC approach to problem-centered learning with its heavy emphasis on active student participation in the
learning process. Most students," according to this opinion, "see medicine as something to know, and therefore that can be taught." (Interview
with a UNM faculty-administrator, 1979.)

Linked to this logic is the opinion that PCC would be most
effective with precisely those students who needed it least: the best and

the brightest. Nevertheless, PCC was accepted as "worth it because of the Hawthorne effect." By this reasoning, the PCC program could be turned around into a faculty-centered program, and if it also somehow accomplished all or some of its stated learner-centered goals, so much the better.

Within PCC itself, there was an atmosphere of orderly chaos, orderly in the intense, purposeful, creative effort that took shape as the PCC cadre raced to get ready for the first group of students who would apply during 1978–1979 and begin studies in the fall of 1979, and chaotic in the rapid changes that were forced upon the planners by the barriers of accreditation in the spring of 1977 and the resource limitations that became evident at the late date of the spring of 1978.

A key factor was the support of Dean Napolitano. The dean, who had been a member of the original faculty of the medical school, supported the program strongly. Although he did not make any judgment ahead of time on its conceptual validity, and even expressed some qualifications about its potential achievement, he believed that PCC should have the fullest possible opportunity to demonstrate its capabilities, and for that purpose, he gave it strong sanction.

These were the conditions under which the final planning of PCC was conducted. There was the security of strategically located support among the leaders of the medical school, coupled with the tensions of a rapidly shifting set of professionally acceptable norms and cost-limited alternatives that were available to the final operational plan. Without being fully aware of it, the founders were fighting to preserve the inner core of values of their original plan and, despite the appearance of support from their colleagues and the success of their grant application to Kellogg, there was trouble stemming from the different perceptions of the meaning of PCC.

In retrospect, it is clear that many of those who supported PCC did so at first from a relatively narrow perspective, looking at it essentially as a program that was oriented toward local problems. In the minds of the founders, on the other hand, the experiment was seen in a much broader perspective. That the issue was not joined until later was due most likely to the decision to introduce PCC into the medical school as an "experiment." Recalling this decision, one of the departmental chairmen said:

"The decision to present the plan for PCC as an experiment was wise. It titillated the academic instincts of our faculty and provided a reversibility to the decision to go ahead with the program, which reassured the skeptics."

Without being fully aware of the fact, the founders of PCC were following a well-trodden path in the history of educational innovations. Faced with the task of introducing a nontraditional mission into an institution that was already vested in a traditional structure, they tempered the potential resistance by creating an enclave within the medical school (Levine, 1980). Such a course allowed for breathing space, the trial period that is so important for new programs. For a McMasters or a Michigan State, the innovative mission becomes part of the establishment of a whole new institution, a much different situation than that which faces the innovator in an already established school.

This then was the atmosphere in which PCC ended its planning stage and entered the first steps of implementation, alive with all the fresh energy of a new idea eager to be tested in action. Despite all the care that had been taken, and the support, it was not long before it faced its first major crisis, an unexpected tension within its leadership.

Division in the Leadership:
A Critical Episode

On that first winter afternoon when Scott Obenshain and Arthur Kaufman shared their disappointments and hopes, they gained only strength and purpose. Working together, they decided, each could be twice as strong, and that is the way it worked, at first. As time passed, however, they discovered other things about each other.

Throughout the first two years, as they defined the educational problem and articulated the plan that was to become the Primary Care Curriculum (PCC), their initial close feeling of collaboration only grew stronger. Although differences in their experience and abilities were always recognized, they complemented each other.

When the planning grant application to the Kellogg Foundation succeeded, however, a turning point was reached, requiring that each should take a more specific, task-directed role. The necessary expansion of effort forced a division of labor. On the one hand, there were all the tasks of preparing specifically for the teaching–learning requirements of problem-based education; and on the other, there were the management and custodial tasks of organizing and sustaining the effort. Faculty development became a separate domain from staff functions. The former tended to fall under the leadership of Kaufman and the latter under Obenshain. It should be emphasized that these were only tendencies. In the egalitarian, sharing atmosphere of the early phases, no such division of labor could be either formal or sharp. Nevertheless, this rough demarcation of responsibility became real enough to shatter the earlier harmony of undifferentiated sharing, and neither the leaders themselves nor the cadre of faculty and staff in the early program team were prepared for it.

The development was gradual. When the first class of ten students arrived in August 1979, PCC began in an atmosphere where the faculty never felt more than one step in front of the students. Although extensive planning had occurred, the methods were so new to everyone involved that the dominant spirit could not be other than improvisational. There were materials ready, but nothing was regarded as permanent and everything was subject to revision. The focus was on the what and how, the content and methods of the program. There were constant meetings to discuss what was happening, to allow all the participants, students, staff, and faculty, to express their feelings about the experience. The theme was problem solving, in all its different varieties. The meetings were to analyze and correct; the notion of failure was not even considered. If something didn't work, it was changed. For the students, the atmosphere was completely nonpunitive and for the faculty the entire emphasis was on quick feedback, correction as you go along, discussion of weakness in order to provide support and help everyone to improve. And everything was egalitarian. Participation in all aspects of the program was allowed according to ability and with no reference to formal qualifications. It was a therapeutic atmosphere. Anything was possible.

This early, self-conscious and purist stage did not last very long. Within a year, the experiment was able to shake down its rough edges and to emerge as an operational program.

By the second year of operation, the central emphasis shifted to questions of feasibility for long-term development. Questions began to be asked about whether and how PCC might be transferred into curriculum for the whole student body. Another important question that was generated concerned the fate of research as a major function if PCC were to be diffused from its experimental status to the curriculum as a whole. These could be interpreted as signs of success. However, instead of creating tensions between PCC and the conventional teaching program, factional divisions occurred inside PCC.

The basic division was between a subsystem whose function was to accomplish specific tasks involved in the teaching program, and a second subsystem which functioned to mediate between task demands and the need to keep the organizational structure in operation. In PCC, the former tended to be thought of as the intellectual and more creative aspects of the work; the latter were seen as program maintenance and custodial requirements. The early minimum division of labor gave way to a tendency to assign management and custodial tasks to people who had no more than a master's degree and, not coincidentally, mainly to women. The program development tasks, on the other hand, began to be concentrated in faculty members of higher rank, mainly those with M.D. or Ph.D. degrees, and these were largely men. Inevitably, different values and rewards were attached to these types of participation. The PCC "family" (as they liked to call themselves) began to divide along traditional lines: the dominant productive roles became primarily a male domain, and the essential but less esteemed "housekeeper" roles, a female domain.

The problems caused by this division of the labor involved more than the leadership. For example, one staff member despite her very junior formal status, had been more responsible for the development of education materials, especially the P4 decks, than anyone else. She was qualified only at the M.A. level as a specialist in education. In the open early phases of the program, her talent, combined with a forthright personality, made her a leader. It seemed natural for her to seek full, creative participation; she asked, for example, to participate as a tutor. In the early egalitarian atmosphere, this wish did not create any conflict. As the program moved toward more structural formality, however, the question of differential qualifications surfaced. Who should be a tutor? it was asked. The answer began to reflect the increased diffusion of PCC into the realm of values for the medical school as a whole. Strong sentiment had developed that only M.D.s or Ph.D.s should be the faculty in the tutorial groups, because the tutorial was the centerpiece of the PCC method.

For a time, this issue was mediated with a compromise: some tutorials were assigned two tutors, one a physician and the other with a different type of degree. The tension remained, however, and in the end this particular staff person, despite her deep attachment to PCC, resigned to take a more highly ranked job at another institution.

Divisions also occurred around differences of approach. There were those who were more radical, more eager to try and to experiment, constantly testing the validity of the original ideas and trying out various ways of accomplishing the objectives. A second group was more cautious, more evolutionary in its approach, and attentive to the normative content in which this already quite radical idea was being tested, willing to at least consider the constraints of the more traditional approaches. Kaufman tended to be perceived as the leader of the more radical group, while Obenshain was the more cautious. Although there were overlapping functions, similar identification of the leaders occurred with the two major subsystems: Kaufman with the task-oriented and Obenshain with the maintenance.

The tension that these divisions generated would normally have been siphoned off by organized group discussions that were designed for just such a purpose, by the catharsis of frank self-appraisal and analysis; and in the beginning that is precisely what occurred. However, as more faculty came into the program, the meetings that brought faculty and staff together disappeared and along with them the regular dialogues between the co-leaders. The tension was deepening until it was brought to the surface by the external consultant on a visit in the fall of 1980. Even then, the full implications of the separation of staff from faculty and of one leader from the other were not faced until the following year, forced again by the external consultant. Only after a full-blown crisis developed around the case of an appointee was any effective remedial action taken.

The Case of John

In 1980, to strengthen the organizational structure of PCC, a grant proposal was written to support a manager of the staff functions. Originally, this position was conceived with a specific person in mind, a woman with demonstrated skills not only in management and administration but in the main purpose of grant writing. When her appointment was proposed, however, it was vetoed by a very highly placed official of the medical school because of a conflict in the history of their professional relations. A young systems analyst was chosen instead, a man with a Ph.D. degree in systems management.

The style of the new appointee (to be called here by the fictional name "John") was bureaucratic. His main duties were defined as the following, listed in the order of their importance:

1. To help conceive and prepare new grant proposals.
2. To organize and oversee the computerization of the numerous data being collected for the internal and external evaluations.
3. To plan the systemization and streamlining of the staff functions.

In operation, he concentrated on the third function. He defined his role by asserting a rigidly formal authority over the staff members and by introducing detailed procedures that codified the management tasks of PCC.

In effect, what John did was to impose a new and unnecessarily detailed system on that part of PCC that was already most efficient. He also exacerbated the already sensitive feelings of individuals who were laboring faithfully in the vineyards but getting what were seen as the least rewards, both materially and intellectually. Moreover, they were a largely feminine group, several of whom were qualified for promotion to leadership, suddenly placed under the authority of a man whose only evident qualification was a higher academic degree.

On a visit in December 1980, the external consultant identified this problem and recommended that the new appointee should be dismissed before a crisis developed. Although both Obenshain and Kaufman agreed with the basic diagnosis of the problem, and the whole matter was brought to the attention of John by the consultant, there was no action taken for another year. In the meantime, Obenshain, who supervised the new position, tried to repair the situation by supporting and retraining John. The result was a deepened division between the factions, with negative feelings focused on John. The resentments of the staff grew, as did tension between the leaders. At one point, the staff began to press for action continuously and even threatened to walk out. Yet the leaders of PCC took no steps to deal with John.

Finally, during a visit of the external consultant in July 1981, the problem was fully discussed in a general meeting of PCC faculty and staff and soon thereafter John was dismissed. By that time, John had been socially isolated and, in effect, he was no longer functioning. Staff operations had reverted to their previous style.

This incident is instructive for several reasons. The most important concerns the balance between personal performance and the structural strains that occur in organizations. Subsystems of production (faculty) and maintenance (staff) are universal in academic organizations. That they should relate to each other in problematic ways is predictable. That leadership divides according to these subsystems is also expected, as is the tendency to fit such leadership assignments with the personal styles of the individuals involved. When problems emerge, the great pitfall is that reaction and interpretation tend to focus on personality. In this case, John was commonly blamed. A different choice, many believed, would have prevented the crisis that occurred. Or the personal style of either Obenshain or Kaufman was seen as the cause. In fact, *the basic conflict was in the structure of the situation.*

PCC was expanding. Both subsystems were enlarged to meet the needs of the increased number of students. As a result, face-to-face meetings of the entire faculty and staff were more cumbersome, and indeed, virtually stopped. Such conditions of expansion and complexity of function in organization typically lead to the rationalization of structure. Bureaucracy, with its hierarchical formal codes of authority and responsibility, is one method to rationalize organization. John tried to bureaucratize PCC. He failed, but not because of his personal style alone. The problems he faced required some form of reorganization. His decisions about how to solve those problems opposed the values of PCC, he communicated poorly, and he failed to win either the sanction of those with more authority or the trust of his subordinates. Even a person with stronger interpersonal skills could have failed in this situation.

Another important lesson to be drawn from this incident concerns the processes of crisis management. The stress that is part of innovation is, in itself, considerable. Just as the innovation is "on trial," so are the innovators. They have taken personal risks, and to be dispassionate and "realistic" when one is in the heat of strenuous creative effort is unlikely. Thus, it was essential to have "outside" consultation, to have a trusted evaluator who observed and reported to the program at regular and short intervals, and who, in effect, was able to assume some of the responsibility for a troublesome, difficult decision.

PCC survived the crisis that centered around John and moved into its third year with its top leadership intact, even strengthened by having successfully negotiated the crisis together. In the meantime, a sub-stratum of leaders had emerged. On the one hand, there was a group of faculty members: two basic scientists, a clinician, an economist. Typically, these individuals began skeptical of the method but attracted by the goals; they were willing to share in the trial. Just as typical was their enthusiastic conversion. For three of them, PCC became a significant factor in major career decisions. When offered important positions in other academic settings, they decided to stay at New Mexico, strongly influenced by their participation in PCC. In the maintenance subsystem, on the other hand, only one new appointment was notable. Characteristically, this was a woman. She defined her role as temporary because her husband was a student who would leave within a finite time period. She, together with the older staff, absorbed John's responsibilities in a quiet, efficient way.

The Crisis of Measurement:
The End of the Experimental Phase

As PCC achieved more and more solid acceptance at the University of New Mexico, the broader educational implications came to the fore. Success as a local program raised consciousness about the generic attributes that could be applied to medical education. Signs of this shift in emphasis appeared as early as November 1980, when the experiences of both students and preceptors in Phase IB, the preceptorship, were reviewed. One of the most striking statements made came from Dr. Thal, a well-known surgeon who was a preceptor in Las Vegas, New Mexico:

> *"What struck me was that I found in this [first-year PCC] student the same aura of joy and pleasure in medicine, in what you are doing, that we all originally believed would be part of doctoring [our emphasis]. This was very different from other, fourth-year medical students who have also worked with me as a preceptor. With these other students, I must say that I was dumbstruck by their almost bovine approach. These students from the regular program seemed to be . . . dulled by overwork or something. Actually, I must say that I at times assumed that this PCC student was a fourth-year student. I certainly was able to communicate with her very easily. I must compliment her. She made it a living, ongoing experience."*

Another preceptor spoke to the same effect:

> *"I went through a family practice residency. By the time I got to it, I had a suppressed distaste for experience in medical school. I am envious of these students. They can learn a lot in a meaningful way. What they are doing seems to start a habit pattern of on-the-job learning as opposed to what I went through. Once you are finished with a block, you are finished. . . ."*

In both of these statements, there is no question that the preceptors are talking about how one becomes a physician, asserting that the PCC approach challenges the validity of the conventional methods by which these preceptors themselves learned. The evaluation team, as early as December 1980, agreed (Bloom & Moore-West, 1980):

> It is the opinion of the evaluation team that the curriculum innovation represented by PCC is a more distinctive change from what has gone before than the PCC conceptualizers themselves yet comprehend. For example, it is sometimes asserted that PCC is a development that has continuity with the curriculum innovations of Western Reserve. We would contend that this comparison is not correct. Western Reserve, in spite of its highly enlightened goals and imaginative reorganization of the curriculum, continues the more traditional emphasis on the content of learning. In effect it maintains the goals of achieving an appropriate *amount of learning,* simply changing the form within which learning accretion occurs. Certainly it tries to make such information relevant, more connected to a coherent and concrete reality in patient care. Nevertheless it maintains the conception that it is *how much one knows* ultimately that determines competency in medicine. PCC, on the other hand, contains a very different orientation. Instead of knowledge

accumulation, it emphasizes the development of the processes of thought that are necessary for individuals to integrate within themselves a sustaining approach to learning.

The same issue can be approached in another way. Medical education, studied as socialization for professional behavior, has documented this conflict between the accumulation of knowledge and learning to solve problems. The issue has been one of memorization versus analysis, obviously not a matter of either/or, but rather a matter of emphasis (Becker et al., 1961; Fox, 1980; Miller, 1980). This persistence of the memorization-mastery of knowledge emphasis in medical education has been observed to have a dulling effect on the intellectual vitality of students and also to blunt their initial idealistic-humanistic value orientation toward the profession. (Bloom, 1978; Funkenstein, 1957, 1971, 1978)

The summary judgment of evaluation at this point in time, two years from the operational beginnings, was that the PCC program was emerging from its trial phase. The analysis by the external evaluators pointed to both the achievements and to hazards, anticipating certain booby traps on the basis of the experience of others. The first was the situation illustrated by the experience with John. Quoting from the evaluation report of July 16 and 23, 1981 (Bloom & Moore-West, 1981):

> PCC is entering a new stage in which pressures to institutionalize are building up. A risk of responding by bureaucratizing . . . should be underscored. Institutionalization does *not* equate with the hierarchical, codified arrangement of authority and responsibility that is represented by bureaucratic organization.

The evaluators' report then turned to a warning based upon experience described in the literature:

> As Miller (1980) reports, such programs (innovations like PCC) repeatedly, after initial success, are deflected from a focus on learning by the perceived need to demonstrate "objectively" that results are congruent with goals. More concretely, examinations are characteristically produced, and such examinations, despite strenuous efforts to diversify their methodology, tend to be memory-centered and therefore to revive the demand for teaching content (measurable) rather than attitudes and behavior skills (hard to measure).
>
> The booby trap is that decisions ultimately are made without reference to such measured success or nonsuccess. Decisions about educational policy are more usually made according to the power factors, especially those related to resource availability. When funding priorities

emphasized science (Sputnik era), the resources for research were the dominant force. Indeed, research has dominated the whole 30-year era; educational ideology was used as a facade to deal with public pressures for the humanization of technology, for blunting the radicalism of the civil rights and war against poverty movements, and for containing community participation.

Thus, even when evidence is provided that supports educational change, the decisions of policymakers are not necessarily directly influenced.

The "measurement" crisis so typical of innovations in medical education did indeed occur in PCC, centered on the National Board— Part I. The performance of PCC students on this examination was quite varied, certainly not as good as had been hoped. Using the NBME as a criterion, a case could have been made against PCC, much as the PCC leaders feared. Instead, different adjustments were made to prepare the PCC students for the Boards. The most recent and most successful is the use of the Shelf Boards, which NBME itself recommends and administers as an interim experience during training and prior to taking the Boards. As a teaching and preparation mechanism, the Shelf Boards are now a standard part of the PCC program.

Was New Mexico's experience different in this respect from that described for Buffalo (Miller, 1980) and Western Reserve (Ham, 1976)? In 1981 it was still too early to tell, even though the first stage of the "measurement crisis" was successfully weathered. There remained the risk that PCC would survive but more in form than in the substance of its ideology.

By July 1981, the external evaluation made the judgment that the experimental phase of PCC was substantially completed. The question now was what would the future role of PCC be?

Pressures for
Institutionalization:
Success? or a
Different Type of Crisis?

By the end of the second year of operation, the site visit report of the external evaluation stated (Bloom & Moore-West, 1981):

The PCC program's position, already trended toward legitimacy earlier than expected six months ago, has continued to move toward operational stability. It is so widely accepted now in the school that the decision about its future status is forced into the foreground of the UNM School of Medicine collective consciousness. (July 16 and 23, 1981)

In the same report, the evaluation asserted that problems of "cost" and "resources" had replaced questions about legitimacy:

> With the experimental phase substantially completed, the competitive position of PCC for the allocation of resources has crystallized as a problem within the medical school. . . . The decision about the future role of PCC has been pushed forward:
> • Will there be a dual-track curriculum?
> • Will PCC become the major teaching mode?
> These questions cannot be ignored. Any estimate of cost, and consequently of cost-effectiveness, rests on these decisions. (Evaluator's Report, July 16 and 23, 1981)

These considerations crystallized in the "F1 hybrid." This was the name given by some of PCC's converts from the basic sciences to the conception of a new curriculum for the whole student body at the University of New Mexico, a curriculum that would include a synthesis of both PCC and conventional-track methods. The leading exponent was Dr. Robert Anderson, the Chairman of the Pathology Department and a highly respected figure in the medical school. His enthusiasm for PCC was stated as follows (personal interview, 1983):

- PCC's first contribution to New Mexico is to drive home the fact that experiments are not only possible with medical education but are essential.
- Second, it has taught select people on the faculty that teaching can be fun again.
- The third aspect is the assignment of the students to positions of responsibility for their own learning.

Moreover, he argued that the adaptation of PCC's basic methodologies for the student body as a whole was feasible for the basic sciences.

Anderson was not content to share and support the work of PCC. He argued that the methodology of PCC should be expanded to include the whole student body of the medical school, and he asserted a leadership role toward that end. He went so far as to compare the evaluation of PCC to a clinical trial. The validity of PCC, in his opinion, had been demonstrated. Therefore, as in the case of successful clinical trials of therapeutic agents, it becomes unethical to withhold access for the population "at risk."

Dr. Anderson was supported in his decision to propose such a decisive step in the history of the New Mexico experiment by the results of a site visit by a select committee of external evaluators created by Dean Napolitano. This committee spent three days observing and reviewing PCC in October 1983. Its members included the following:

Parker A. Small, Jr., M.D., Professor of Immunology and Medical Microbiology and Professor of Pediatrics, University of Florida, Gainesville.

Hilliard Jason, M.D., E.D.D., National Center for Faculty Development in the Health Professions, University of Miami School of Medicine.

Ascher Segall, M.D., Director, Center for Educational Development in Health, Boston University.

Carmine D. Clemente, Professor and Chairman, Department of Anatomy, University of California at Los Angeles.

Anthony Imbembo, M.D., Professor of Surgery, Western Reserve University School of Medicine.

The visit of this committee served as a stimulus for PCC to distill the most essential description and analysis of its work and achievements into a condensed summary form. The committee itself observed and interviewed, looking closely at all possible aspects of the program. The result was a gratifyingly strong endorsement of PCC. Although the judgments were by no means uniform, their conclusion was unmistakable. They saw PCC as a teaching–learning experiment which had, with clearly articulated goals, changed the experience of its students in a manner that was appropriate to the practice of medicine in the future. With the exception of only one member of this committee, the visitors were not merely approving, they were excited. They also judged the accomplishment as appropriate to the teaching of scientific information. Not only was this an educational approach that was relevant to clinical medicine, but they found it effective for the transmission of scientific reasoning and research skills.

It was striking that the emphasis of the committee was on the nature of the teaching–learning experience. In terms of professional outcomes, the manpower goals of the program, little was said. The heavy emphasis was on the quality of education and the intrinsic processes of teaching–learning.

Against this background, it was all the more possible for Dr. Anderson to propose to the New Mexico faculty a new approach to medical education for the whole school:

"*The University of New Mexico has developed and implemented a separate learner-centered, problem-based learning group curricular track over the past five years. Although this effort has been successful, components of the experimental curriculum are difficult for faculty at other medical schools to perceive as an answer to their educational problems. We will take components of this innovative track, adapt and modify them to meet the perceived needs of faculty, and combine them with innovations occurring elsewhere in higher education. This will then become the major curriculum at the University of New Mexico School of Medicine and will serve as a template which can be more easily adapted, all or part, to other medical schools. It will activate the learner, decrease the adversarial relationships between students and faculty, raise the level of cognitive function of students. . . .*"

One of the most striking aspects of the Anderson proposal is its full conversion of PCC's values to a universal frame of reference. Virtually no mention is made of the particular local goals of PCC as a New Mexico program. The whole thrust is to extract "the basic educational philosophy of the program, i.e., learner-centered and problem-based." In effect, Anderson is proposing the most radical direction of all, that is, to establish a paradigm for all of medical education based upon the lessons and intrinsic core of PCC.

Within this current situation there is much anxiety about the fate of PCC as an ideology. If there is an Fl hybrid created, the PCC faculty who are most devoted to the central values of the program worry that there will be a corruption of the processes of learning as they are now structured by PCC. This is an opinion that was strongly presented by one of the members of the select committee of external evaluators: Hilliard Jason. He recommended in the most forceful terms that PCC should be continued as a separate track. His reasoning was that this offered a unique opportunity in the history of medical education to have a longitudinal program of research to monitor the differential effects of this very innovative and important type of education compared with the more conventional medical education.

Testing a Model of
Educational Innovation

A recent model of innovation in higher education (Levine, 1980) suggests a useful frame of reference for the interpretation of PCC. An innovation is operationally defined as any departure from the traditional practices of an organization. The key words are "new" and "different," the combination of the elements of reform and change, "reform" implying new and "change" implying different (Levine, 1980:3–4). The process of innovation, Levine asserts, involves a series of predictable, sequential stages. This general proposition is not unique to Levine (Hage & Aiken, 1970; Mann & Neff, 1961; Rogers & Shoemaker, 1971; Smelser, 1959). However, Levine's model is based on the closest analogue to the subject of this study, that is, the introduction of a new program in an institution of higher learning; and although it is not specific to medical education, we believe that it applies. The stages of Levine's model are as follows:

1. Recognizing the need for change—it is realized that some organizational need is not being satisfied.
2. Planning and formulating a means of satisfying the need—a concrete plan is developed.
3. Initiating and implementing the plan—the plan is put into operation on a trial basis.
4. Institutionalizing or terminating the new operating plan—either the operating plan is routinized and integrated into the organization or it is ended. (Levine, 1980:6–7)

Concerning the origins of educational innovations, Levine attributes the most significance to environmental conditions. We have seen how both the national social climate and the local state opinion in 1976 showed deep concern about the distribution of medical manpower and the lack of primary care (Chapter 1). Similar needs are reflected in international organizations, such as the WHO-sponsored "Network of Community-Oriented Educational Institutions for Health Sciences.

We have described how PCC carried through the first three steps of this model, arriving at the present stage of institutionalization. Its method was to create what Levine calls an "innovative enclave within an existing college." Such enclaves are designed to reduce anxiety and fear of general change, but there are risks:

The disadvantages of enclaves are that they can become appendages isolated from the rest of the campus, sanctuaries for dissatisfied faculty and students, and a means of preventing an institution from making needed institutional changes. (Levine, 1980:5)

Such risk is increased when an institution possesses a strong organizational identity. Organizations, like individual persons, "guard their personalities against entropic forces" (Levine, 1980:11).

To change the whole organization, there must be a change in the organization's norms, values, and goals. This can occur only when "environmental change makes existing boundaries unworkable, when the organization fails to achieve desired goals, or when it is thought that goals can better be satisfied in another manner" (Levine, 1980:12). The use of an enclave hedges the organizational bets. It allows the testing of the innovation without tampering with the organization's norms. Eventually, experience indicates, there must be a resolution of the inherent contradiction of such a situation.

> The presence of two separate and divergent boundary systems combines to provide multiple or blurred definitions of organizational character. An organization cannot function in this manner because each boundary system pulls it in a different direction. (Levine, 1980:14)

In the case of PCC, the school's acceptance initially signified only that the advantages were perceived to outweigh the risks. As the planning stage ended with the academic year 1978–1979, the experiment was in place, a bounded system within another very different system. By 1983, the pressure for congruence replaced the "moratorium."

To deal with the conflict between host and enclave, Levine proposes two mechanisms:

> The first mechanism is called *boundary expansion* and involves the adoption of the innovation's personality traits by the host, or more simply an acceptance by the host of some or all of the innovation's differences. Owing to the dominant position of the organization, there is very rarely a complete acceptance of innovation differences; far more common are mutual changes in both host and innovation personalities, agreed upon by joint negotiation and resulting in a *hybridization* of the two (our emphasis). (Levine, 1980:14)

This is the process that Levine calls boundary diffusion. The second mechanism is called *boundary contraction* and involves "a constriction of organizational boundaries in such a manner as to exclude innovation differences" (Levine, 1980:14). Obviously the latter does not apply in the case of PCC, while diffusion and its "hybridization" do.

Summary

In this chapter, we have attempted to trace the processes whereby PCC, as an innovation in medical education, moved from an experimental to an accepted successful local program at the University of New Mexico. We have attempted to show with illustrations the challenges that occur in such a course, but more importantly the attempt has been made to trace the patterns of PCC's development and to relate them to a model that describes stages of innovation in higher education. The result reveals that, in broad outline, the experiences of PCC follow patterns that are more characteristic of general experience than they are unique. This detracts not at all from the contribution that PCC makes to medical education. It merely points out that there are certain patterns in the process of developing new educational programs that are predictable. A clear portrait of these patterns helps us to understand why PCC has continued to succeed and establish itself both in the consciousness and structure of UNM and as an example of an educational ideology and method on a broader scale in medical education. It also helps to clarify the nature and source of the tensions, pressures, conflicts, and crises experienced during the first five years of PCC and to explain how its practitioners have managed to resolve most of its basic problems.

Despite its evident success, the full test of PCC is yet to come. The challenge, it becomes increasingly clear, is a fundamental one. What is known as "the conventional track" at New Mexico is much more than that. It is a coherent, long-standing approach to medical education that has dominated American medical schools for 75 years. Can PCC successfully challenge such an established ideology and educational methodology? Seeking the answer to this question, it is necessary first to understand what the fundamental nature of that challenge actually is.

On the surface, PCC appears to represent an attempt to bring into clearer focus learning for physicianhood in medical education. As such, it represents a shift from the domination by research in American medical education since the so-called Flexner revolution. The irony in the PCC experience has been its appeal to basic scientists even while, on the surface, its approach was at first perceived by some to be a threat to the research orientation of conventional approaches to medical education.

One explanation is that beneath the emphasis on more effective teaching methodology, there is inherent in the PCC process a model for scientific reasoning. By comparison, the marriage between research science and conventional medical education was more a matter of power structure than it was an integrated representation of the values of science in the teaching–learning model. More concretely, it is our judgment that medical education has been dominated by premises that were valid in 1920 but which were obsolete by 1950. That is, in 1920 it was important to make sure that students, most of whom came to medical school relatively poorly prepared, were drilled in the basics. By 1950, this was no longer true; students came to medical school much better prepared in the basics and more oriented toward science.

In the meantime, science as an enterprise was institutionalized in medical schools even while the teaching was not very compatible with the methods of science. Problem solving and an emphasis on decision making are the true essence of scientific reasoning. But the conventional curriculum tended to be so content-oriented that students were overwhelmed by the requirements of memorization. In this situation, didactic teaching was convenient for a faculty that needed as much time as possible for its research and therefore wanted to limit its involvement in the time-consuming demands of sensitive communication in teaching.

PCC brings the problem into a clearer perspective. The scientists who participate in PCC are very excited by what they find in the teaching–learning process. They find students learning in just the ways that are most exciting to them in the work of science. Suddenly, no matter what the amount of teaching time involved, they are excited by what they are doing because it is familiar to them and part of their commitment as scientists.

The paradox then becomes one essentially of vested power. Can one change a coherent structure such as is represented by the conventional patterns of American medical education, even though one has a demonstrated model that more effectively teaches both for scientific and clinical reasoning?

References

Becker, H. S., Geer, B., Hughes, E. C., & Strauss, A. M. (1961). *Boys in white, student cultures in medical school.* Chicago: University of Chicago Press.

Bloom, S. W. (1973). *Power and dissent in the medical school.* New York: The Free Press of Macmillan.

Bloom, S. W. (1978). Socialization for the physician's role: A review of some contributions of research to theory. In E. C. Shapiro & L. M. Lowenstein (Eds.), *Becoming a physician* (pp. 3–52). Cambridge, Mass.: Ballinger.

Bloom, S. W., & Moore-West, M. (Dec. 1980). Interim external evaluator's report to PCC No. 1. Primary Care Curriculum, University of New Mexico School of Medicine.

Bloom, S. W., & Moore-West, M. (July, 1981). Interim external evaluator's report to PCC No. 2. Primary Care Curriculum, University of New Mexico School of Medicine.

Fox, R. C. (1980). *Essays in medical sociology.* New York: Wiley–Interscience.

Funkenstein, D. H. (1957). Possible contributions of psychological testing of the nonintellectual characteristics of medical school applicants. In H. H.Gee & J. T. Cowles (Eds.), *The appraisal of applicants to medical school* (pp. 88–112). Evanston, Ill.: The Association of American Colleges.

Funkenstein, D. H. (1971). Medical students, medical schools and society during three eras. In R. H. Coombs & C. E. Vincent (Eds.), *Psychosocial aspects of medical training* (pp. 229–284). Springfield, Ill.: Charles C. Thomas.

Funkenstein, D. H. (1978). *Medical students, medical schools, and society during five eras.* Cambridge, Mass.: Ballinger.

Hage, J., & Aiken, M. (1970). *Social change in complex organizations.* New York: Random House.

Ham, T. H. (1976). *The student as colleague: Medical education experience at Western Reserve.* Ann Arbor: University Microfilms International.

Levine, A. (1980). *Why innovation fails.* Albany: State University of New York Press.

Mann, F., & Neff, F. W. (1961). *Managing major change in organizations.* Ann Arbor: Foundation for Research on Human Behavior.

Miller, G. (1980). *Training medical educators.* Cambridge, Mass.: Harvard University Press.

Moss, J. Z. (1970). Concurrent evaluation: An approach to action research. *Social Science and Medicine, 4* (Suppl. 1), 25–30.

Rogers, E., & Shoemaker, F. F. (1971). *Communication of innovations.* New York: Free Press.

Smelser, N. (1959). *Social change in the industrial revolution: An application of theory to the Lancashire Cotton Industry.* Chicago: University of Chicago Press.

CHAPTER 14

Reflections

ARTHUR KAUFMAN

As I reflect on the last eight years of the planning and implementation of PCC, I see a maturing of the program's educational ideas. The early, frenetic activity of proposing, debating, and defending competing educational approaches has given way to a general consensus around a core of underlying values. These values, discussed below, have emerged from the testing ground of student and faculty experience.

Student-Centered Learning Is
More a Value Than a Method

When PCC began, our faculty and staff were wed to a series of problem-based tutorial *methods* modified from other institutions. These methods were consistent with the goals for our students, emphasizing reasoning and group interaction. We thought that if we were faithful to the methods, the goals could be achieved.

Suggesting the slightest deviation from the codified methods caused ripples of anxiety throughout the program. Yet, in retrospect, the many changes in methods undertaken by PCC over the years were consistent with the underlying *values* of the program. Although these values have been expressed in numerous ways, they have remained unwritten. What are they?

1. Students are the best judges of the quality and effectiveness of their own education. The best ideas in education will emerge

from paying careful attention to the students—what they do, what they say, and what they feel. The program should be adjusted accordingly.

2. The social status that usually separates teachers from students inhibits learning. Student-centered learning minimizes these obstacles, liberating students and faculty alike to approach each problem cooperatively.

3. An optimum learning environment is one in which students and faculty are excited about their educational activities. When both are participants in learning, analyzing problems, and drawing conclusions, each reaps benefits. If students are bored or faculty is uninterested, there is something drastically wrong.

4. Competitiveness between students is a destructive force in education when it replaces mutual support and caring. The tutorial process can have a strong influence in promoting helping attitudes, which should be the hallmark of a physician.

Control over Student Evaluation Symbolizes the Conflict between Student-Centered and Teacher-Centered Learning

PCC put its major investment in the quality of students' learning rather than in the rigor of its student evaluation. In fact, we believed that some of the most important learning in medical school is least amenable to numerical evaluation. This quickly surfaced as a major clash of values underlying the attitudes of faculty in the two tracks. As one astute observer of the medical education scene has noted,

> Some very dubious educational practices are excused on the grounds that they are *maintaining standards*, or even, Lord help us, raising standards. It is too often assumed that one maintains or defends educational standards by setting up complex and difficult examinations, preferably with a high failure rate. A public-health equivalent to this concept would be interesting. We would institute a public-health screening program, so adjusting the normal values that a large proportion of the population would fail to pass as fit. We could then shake our heads, sad, but confident that we had raised the standards of public health (Simpson, 1974).

In the early years we failed to appreciate fully the degree of importance faculty in a teacher-centered curriculum attribute to their control over student evaluation. It is a cornerstone of their power over students, their legitimacy, the symbol and expression of the expert knowledge they possess. Sadly, it is a hollow legitimacy which consumes an inordinate amount of faculty time. This time could be spent more profitably in modeling for students the faculty's real expertise—a scientific approach to problems. Faculty could also make a more long-lasting contribution to their students' future by facilitating students' gradual assumption of responsibility for evaluating their own learning.

In a lecture-based program most students are anonymous. The teacher cannot sense whether students are mastering the material presented. The examination thus becomes the benchmark of student learning. Unfortunately, if students do poorly on the test, the tendency is to blame the student, maintain the identical educational format, and simply recycle the student through it. However, in a problem-based, tutorial program, the students are observed and challenged at close range, and a clearer sense of their strengths and weaknesses emerges. This permits an accurate narrative evaluation to be made and more specific remediation to be arranged. However, to conventional faculty, narrative evaluation of a student seems soft and imprecise.

The real, underlying issue emerged more clearly when PCC decided to employ the National Board of Medical Examiners—Part I, the "gold standard" of many conventional faculty, as one of the routine evaluation instruments for PCC students. This muted criticism of PCC student evaluation temporarily, but after a grace period of quiet grumbling, a number of conventional faculty began to protest that "National Boards aren't a good enough evaluation instrument."

The underlying issue was never really the level of PCC students' performance after all. It was a matter of control: who controls student evaluation? Teacher-centered faculty do not want to defer to national examinations or to some tutor in PCC who isn't even expert in the areas in which he is tutoring. Such traditional faculty are even more incredulous that PCC relinquishes so much control of student evaluation to the students themselves. PCC was a very large threat to a strongly entrenched value system.

The solution to this clash of values has evolved by inviting these very same critics to take part in the program—to tutor in PCC. After tutoring many find that PCC is no longer an abstract and ill-conceived idea, but a valuable program which has provided them with an important, personal experience. New tutors soon grasp the value of student-centered learning as a force for liberating creativity and responsibility on the part of students, and they seem more willing to loosen their grip on a tight control of student evaluation. Students seem to them more trustworthy. Some new faculty are even willing to share control of evaluation with students.

The Community Is an
Extraordinary Environment for
Problem-Based Learning

PCC planners underestimated the power of the community-based phases of the program as a problem-based learning environment. Originally conceived as a strategy to interest students in rural primary care, they have emerged as the strongest challenge to students' clinical reasoning and integration of learning resources. In the community there are no simulations, no paper cases. In the community students must confront patient problems in all their complexity, learning to consider not only the patient's presenting problem but the pertinent family, community, and environmental influences.

Students who have worked in the community in a sustained, productive manner seem altered by this experience and view their education and subsequent hospital clerkships differently. They feel more self-assured, reflective, and resilient on the wards. Their confidence is higher, and they have a better grasp of the broad potential of practice options after formal education. They also have confronted the strong social, political, and economic forces that underlie much of the illness seen in a doctor's office.

PCC has seen the community experience as a testing ground for the degree of maturity and responsibility students are able to assume over their own learning. The community thus adds a vital dimension to our understanding of a student's capabilities. What seemed minor problems on campus can become magnified in the community. On the other hand, students who are quieter or less adept at the intense interactions in tutorials very often blossom when they work more independently under different circumstances in the community.

The results of using community-based education as a vehicle to draw faculty out of their ivory towers, so they can better appreciate the challenges and complexity of community practice, have been very impressive. Faculty also become fully aware that their educational ideas must eventually be translated by the student into the reality of a physician's practice. The town–gown dichotomy fades as faculty and community physicians build a personal relationship around a common concern for a student they share. Extensive community-based learning can thus ignite changes among the medical center faculty. The university can learn to become a better partner and resource for the state's practicing physicians.

Program Adaptability and
Responsiveness are Key Virtues

PCC has created a framework in which program modification and rapid response to student and faculty concerns are institutionalized. The value of this climate cannot be overemphasized, for it fosters strong feelings of program ownership among participants. It also generates an ambience that is most likely to liberate the broadest possible creativity in educational endeavors.

When faculty members who had not been a part of the original planning of PCC began to work in the program, the program improved. They brought newer ideas—such as problem-based approaches to the gross anatomy experience, dog physiology laboratories, and tutorial approaches to pathology case conferences. Owing to our early insecurities, we resisted such suggestions because they didn't fit our preconceived notions. As a consequence we appeared somewhat elitist and doctrinaire, alienating those who could have contributed so much.

By keeping the structure somewhat loose and flexible, PCC is also able to adapt to the unique and varied learning needs of its students. Students learn in different ways. They vary in study patterns, degree of openness in groups, and ability to excel in independent study. A problem-based learning program can foster its own dogma and create its own rigid constraints, and this must be guarded against. The value of tailored learning can be undermined by blind adherence to particular methods.

As we have opened the door to newer approaches, we have learned a great deal about our own abilities to change and grow and to partake of the richness that others have to offer.

Personal Experience with
Problem-Based Learning Is the
Cornerstone of Successful
Recruitment to the Method

When PCC began, we underestimated the importance of the faculty's personal contact with the program, especially with its students, as a determinant of their attitudes toward problem-based learning. We channeled too much energy into arguing the theoretical merits of the method. We relied on our students' high test scores and superior ward evaluations to win faculty converts to the cause. But we found that the conversion came, instead, as faculty "lived" with students in tutorial groups.

The same faculty member who makes decisions by weighing data scientifically at the workbench now makes decisions on the basis of tradition, politics, and anecdote when he enters the world of education. Thus most faculty members will warm to problem-based learning, not because educational research validates its methods, but because of the joy they experience in stimulating their students to seek and discover, rather than simply to sit and absorb. The importance of the experience is enhanced by the camaraderie they feel with faculty from very different disciplines who are drawn together around a common idea in education.

The Value of Problem-Based
Learning Is Not Easily Documented

I wish we had worried less about how PCC students compared with their conventional-track peers and relished more the relevance of the experiences they were having, the excitement they felt about their education, and the success with which they were winning faculty over to their program. Can we show that graduates of problem-based learning programs are "better"? While I think almost all students who go through such a program have received a broader, more relevant education than had they gone the traditional route, I suspect that this assertion is virtually impossible to prove. We do not have the instruments to test the hypothesis, and the students are far too complex and unpredictable to ascribe results to any particular variables.

It is difficult to know which results are attributable to personality, which to prior experience, which to extracurricular influences, and which to problem-based learning itself. Our recent attempt to randomize applicants into PCC is a gesture in the interests of clean experimental design, but even here the unknown variables may be substantial.

Problem-Based Tutorial
Learning Is Cost-Effective

At the very time PCC was becoming increasingly accepted within the medical school as an educational alternative, rising economic uncertainty was forcing all academic programs to consider freezing or reducing budgets. PCC planners were worried. At first glance, problem-based learning in small groups seems more costly in terms of faculty time than traditional, lecture-based education. Thus, PCC planners increasingly feared that the costliness of the program would prove to be its Achilles heel.

This fear proved to be unfounded. Although running two educational tracks *is* more costly, problem-based, tutorial learning was found to require almost the same faculty time per student as conventional education. Further, a research and development track can attract educational grants that more than pay for its cost. Even more important, problem-based tutorial learning sharply increases faculty–student contact time as it reduces preparation time.

When one adds to this the educational benefits to faculty and students in the intellectually stimulating environment of a tutorial group, and the benefits to communities of this form of education, the benefit/cost ratio increases even further.

* * * * * *

Whatever lessons one can draw from the University of New Mexico experience must be tempered by the following considerations:

1. We have a relatively small student body.
2. We began PCC in a social environment in which legislative pressure existed for the medical school to address rural, primary care, manpower needs.
3. Though the University of New Mexico School of Medicine was a well-established institution by the time PCC began, it had not yet become encumbered with such strong traditions that one could not undertake a major experiment in medical education.

We cannot make recommendations about implementing problem-based learning which could be incorporated, cookbook fashion, into other medical schools. Each institution is unique and cannot accept adoption of New Mexico's methods *en bloc*. However, by providing the rich detail of our experience, and touching upon some of the important innovations at other problem-based schools, we hope readers can select those aspects that will be most adaptable to their own environments.

Reference

Simpson, M. A. (1974, March 9). A mythology of medical education. *Lancet*, pp. 399–401.

Index

Index

Springer publishing company

From the Springer Series on
Medical Education

How to Design a Problem-Based Curriculum for the Preclinical Years
Howard S. Barrows
Describes the full range of tasks required in order to implement a successful problem-based curriculum. Thoroughly explains this dynamic, intellectually involved learning approach. 160pp / 1985

Problem-Based Learning
An Approach to Medical Education
Howard Barrows and Robin Tamblyn
"Problem-based learning is defined as self-instruction using patient, health delivery, or research problems to stimulate learning. The arguments are well presented ... excellent, stimulating."—*The Lancet.* 224pp / 1980

The Art of Teaching Primary Care
Golden, Carlson, Hagen, Editors
Details the rationale, structure, and methods used in the education of community-based primary care practitioners. "The innovative, often unorthodox efforts of the authors and their colleagues proved to be an exciting way to train health professionals."—*American Journal of Public Health.* 368pp / 1981

Teaching Preventive Medicine in Primary Care
William Barker, Editor
Prominent educators address diverse issues related to prevention training for future clinicians. "Complete, up-to-date, and extremely well organized." —*Continuing Education for the Family Physician.* 336pp / 1983

Assessing Clinical Competence
Victor Neufeld and Geoffrey Norman, Editors
A comprehensive and critical review of methods used to evaluate competence in the health professions, with attention to the implications of these insights for education, licensing, further research, and service delivery. 384pp / 1984

The Interpersonal Dimension in Medical Education
Agnes Rezler and Joseph Flaherty
Presents up-to-date findings on the importance of personal attitudes, values, and communication skills in the doctor-patient relationship, and describes how this interaction can be promoted through student selection and admission practices. 240pp / 1984

Order from your bookdealer or directly from publisher.
Springer Publishing Co. 536 Broadway, New York, NY 10012

Springer publishing company

Geriatrics and the Law
Patient Rights and Professional Responsibilities
Marshall Kapp and **Arthur Bigot**
Examines every aspect of geriatrics practice from a legal viewpoint: health-care financing, involuntary commitment, guardianship, powers of attorney, informed consent, and more. Explains complex medicolegal issues in clear, easy-to-understand language. 272pp / 1984

Vitalizing Long-Term Care
The Teaching Nursing Home and Other Perspectives
Stuart F. Spicker and **Stanley R. Ingman**
This interdisciplinary volume advocates a new spirit in long-term care emphasizing service, teaching, and research. A key element in this strategy is geriatric training for all medical students. 256pp / 1984

Aging and Public Health
Harry Phillips and **Susan Gaylord,** Editors
This unique text answers the need for a full evaluation of the practice of gerontology from a public health perspective. This involves essential services in health, housing, nutrition, community resources, and other areas of vital concern. Also examined are biological, environmental, and psychosocial aspects and their implications for public health. 1985

Depression and Aging
Causes, Care, and Consequences
Lawrence Breslau and **Marie Haug,** Editors
The social, psychological, nutritional, and organic causes of depression; methods of treatment; and the social and economic consequences. 352pp / 1983

Geriatric Diagnostics
A Case Study Approach
Lucille Nahemow and **Lidia Pousada**
Explores the medical, psychological, and social factors that influence geriatric disorders and their management. "The clinician who is to deliver optimal care must integrate humane and interpersonal qualities in the treatment process. 'Geriatric Diagnostics' plays a valuable role in clarifying this approach." — from the foreword by Carl Eisdorfer. "Highly recommended for students." — *Annals of Internal Medicine.* 352pp / 1983

Geriatric Medicine for the Primary Care Practitioner
Edward B. Elkowitz
A concise overview of the medical problems of geriatric patients, from the perspective of the family practitioner. "An important addition to geriatric literature. It serves as source material for medical student and practitioner alike." — *Journal of the American Osteopathic Association.* 240pp / 1981

Order from your bookdealer or directly from publisher.
Springer Publishing Co. 536 Broadway, New York, NY 10012

Springer publishing company

Introduction to Environmental Health
Daniel Blumethal, Editor

A complete overview, including such key issues as hazardous waste management, occupational health, infectious agents, and radiation dangers. Recommended as a text for students of medicine, nursing, and public health. 272pp / 1985

Cancer Treatment and Research in Humanistic Perspective
Steven Gross and **Solomon Garb,** Editors
Foreword: **R. Lee Clark**

A forum of views on the pressing humanistic concerns that accompany the onset and treatment of cancer. Discusses drug experimentation, ineffective therapies, pain treatment, psychosocial problems, needs of cancer-care professionals, and more. 256pp / 1985

Critical Issues in Family Practice
Cases and Commentaries
Kenneth Kushner, Harry Mayhew, Leroy Rodgers, Rita Hermann, Editors

This stimulating text presents incidents of difficult professional, ethical, and emotional dilemmas faced by family physicians and physicians-in-training. 270pp / 1982

Chronic Illness and Disability through the Life Span
Effects on Self and Family
Myron G. Eisenberg, LaFaye C. Sutkin,
and **Mary A. Jansen,** Editors

This text combines developmental and family systems perspectives to examine the impact of chronic and disabling conditions on the individual within the family context. Original articles written especially for this volume by prominent professionals describe the problems and capacities involved in coping with disability at each life stage. 1984

Advances in Disease Prevention
Charles Arnold, Editor

Integrates new findings in preventive care to provide a basis for patient teaching and guidance at all levels of health care, with an emphasis on chronic illness such as hypertension and heart disease. 320pp / 1981

Hospice Approaches to Pediatric Care
Charles Corr and **Donna Corr,** Editors

Brings to the care of children the principles of the hospice movement, with an emphasis on home care and maximization of quality of life. Includes approaches to chronic conditions, terminal illnesses, and the experience of bereavement. 304pp / 1985

Order from your bookdealer or directly from publisher.
Springer Publishing Co. 536 Broadway, New York, NY 10012